Therapeutic Hotline: New Developments in Dermatology

Editor

SEEMAL R. DESAI

DERMATOLOGIC CLINICS

www.derm.theclinics.com

Consulting Editor
BRUCE H. THIERS

April 2019 • Volume 37 • Number 2

ELSEVIER

1600 John F. Kennedy Boulevard • Suite 1800 • Philadelphia, Pennsylvania, 19103-2899

http://www.theclinics.com

DERMATOLOGIC CLINICS Volume 37, Number 2
April 2019 ISSN 0733-8635, ISBN-13: 978-0-323-68236-7

Editor: Jessica McCool
Developmental Editor: Sara Watkins

Dermatologic Clinics (ISSN 0733-8635) is published quarterly by Elsevier Inc., 360 Park Avenue South, New York, NY 10010-1710. Months of publication are January, April, July, and October. Business and editorial offices: 1600 John F. Kennedy Blvd., Suite 1800, Philadelphia, PA 19103-2899. Customer service office: 11830 Westline Drive, St. Louis, MO 63146. Periodicals postage paid at New York, NY, and additional mailing offices. Subscription prices are USD 404.00 per year for US individuals, USD 736.00 per year for US institutions, USD 456.00 per year for Canadian individuals, USD 898.00 per year for Canadian institutions, USD 510.00 per year for international individuals, USD 898.00 per year for international institutions, USD 100.00 per year for US students/residents, and USD 240.00 per year for Canadian and international students/residents. International air speed delivery is included in all *Clinics* subscription prices. All prices are subject to change without notice. **POSTMASTER:** Send address changes to *Dermatologic Clinics*, Elsevier Health Sciences Division, Subscription Customer Service, 3251 Riverport Lane, Maryland Heights, MO 63043. **Customer Service: 1-800-654-2452 (U.S. and Canada); 314-447-8871 (outside U.S. and Canada). Fax: 314-447-8029. E-mail: journalscustomerservice-usa@elsevier.com (for print support); journalsonlinesupport-usa@elsevier.com (for online support).**

Reprints. For copies of 100 or more, of articles in this publication, please contact the Commercial Reprints Department, Elsevier Inc., 360 Park Avenue South, New York, New York 10010-1710. Tel.: 212-633-3874; Fax: 212-633-3820; Email: reprints@elsevier.com.

The *Dermatologic Clinics* is covered in *MEDLINE/PubMed (Index Medicus), Current Contents/Clinical Medicine, Excerpta Medica, Chemical Abstracts,* and *ISI/BIOMED.*

Contributors

CONSULTING EDITOR

BRUCE H. THIERS, MD
Professor and Chairman Emeritus, Department of Dermatology and Dermatologic Surgery, Medical University of South Carolina, Charleston, South Carolina, USA

EDITOR

SEEMAL R. DESAI, MD, FAAD
Founder & Medical Director, Innovative Dermatology, Havertown, Pennsylvania, USA; Clinical Assistant Professor, Department of Dermatology, The University of Texas Southwestern Medical Center, Dallas, Texas, USA

AUTHORS

CHRISTINE AHN, MD
Department of Dermatology, Wake Forest School of Medicine, Wake Forest University, Winston-Salem, North Carolina, USA

AHMED ANSARI, BS
University of Central Florida, College of Medicine, Orlando, Florida, USA

HILARY E. BALDWIN, MD
Medical Director, The Acne Treatment and Research Center, Morristown, New Jersey, USA; Clinical Associate Professor of Dermatology, Rutgers Robert Wood Johnson Medical Center, New Brunswick, New Jersey, USA

EMMA GUTTMAN-YASSKY, MD, PhD
Vice Chair for Research and Professor of Dermatology, Department of Dermatology, Laboratory for Inflammatory Skin Diseases, Icahn School of Medicine at Mount Sinai, New York, New York, USA

ILTEFAT HAMZAVI, MD
Department of Dermatology, Henry Ford Hospital System, Detroit, Michigan, USA

CALLIE R. HILL, BS
University of Alabama at Birmingham School of Medicine, Birmingham, Alabama, USA

WILLIAM C. HUANG, MD, MPH
Department of Dermatology, Wake Forest School of Medicine, Wake Forest University, Winston-Salem, North Carolina, USA

KHALAF KRIDIN, MD, PhD
Department of Dermatology, Rambam Health Care Campus, Haifa, Israel

MARK LEBWOHL, MD
Waldman Professor and Chair of the Kimberly and Eric J. Waldman Department of Dermatology, Icahn School of Medicine at Mount Sinai, New York, New York, USA

HENRY W. LIM, MD
Chair Emeritus, Department of Dermatology,
Henry Ford Medical Center, Detroit, Michigan,
USA

ALEXIS B. LYONS, MD
Department of Dermatology, Henry Ford
Hospital System, Detroit, Michigan, USA

AUSTIN J. MADDY, BA
Department of Dermatology and Cutaneous
Surgery, University of Miami Miller School of
Medicine, Miami, Florida, USA

JUSTIN W. MARSON, BA
Medical Student IV, Rutgers Robert Wood
Johnson Medical School, Piscataway, New
Jersey, USA

**LEOPOLDO DUAILIBE NOGUEIRA
SANTOS, MD**
Dermatologist, Department of Medicine,
University of Taubaté, Santa Casa of São Paulo
School of Medicine, Municipal Public Servant
Hospital of São Paulo, São Paulo, Brazil

ANJELICA PEACOCK, BS
Wayne State University School of Medicine,
Detroit, Michigan, USA

GISELLE PRADO, MD
Clinical Research Fellow, National Society for
Cutaneous Medicine, New York, New York,
USA

YAEL RENERT-YUVAL, MD
Attending Dermatologist and Clinical
Instructor, Department of Dermatology,
Hadassah-Hebrew University Medical Center,
Hadassah Ein-Kerem Medical Center,
Jerusalem, Israel

DARRELL S. RIGEL, MD, MS
Clinical Professor, Department of
Dermatology, NYU School of Medicine, New
York, New York, USA

NAVEED SAMI, MD
Department of Medicine, University of Central
Florida, Health Sciences Campus at Lake
Nona, Orlando, Florida, USA

JERRY SHAPIRO, MD, FAAD, FRCP
Professor, Ronald O. Perelman Department
of Dermatology, New York University
School of Medicine, New York,
New York, USA

RYAN M. SVOBODA, MD, MS
Clinical Research Fellow, Department
of Dermatology, Duke University
School of Medicine, Durham,
North Carolina, USA

AMY THEOS, MD
Director, Associate Professor, Department
of Dermatology, University of Alabama
at Birmingham, Birmingham, Alabama,
USA

ANTONELLA TOSTI, MD
Department of Dermatology and Cutaneous
Surgery, University of Miami Miller School of
Medicine, Miami, Florida, USA

GAUTHAM VELLAICHAMY, BS
Department of Dermatology,
Henry Ford Hospital System, Wayne State
University School of Medicine, Detroit,
Michigan, USA

STEPHANIE VON CSIKY-SESSOMS
Medical Student IV, Icahn School of
Medicine at Mount Sinai, New York,
New York, USA

ALBERT C. YAN, MD, FAAP, FAAD
Chief, Section of Dermatology, Children's
Hospital of Philadelphia, Professor,
Pediatrics and Dermatology, Perelman
School of Medicine at the University of
Pennsylvania, Philadelphia,
Pennsylvania, USA

DANIELLE G. YEAGER, MD
Resident Physician, Department of
Dermatology, Henry Ford Medical Center,
Detroit, Michigan, USA

RAHEEL ZUBAIR, MD, MHS
Department of Dermatology, Henry Ford
Hospital System, Detroit, Michigan,
USA

Contents

choices. Spironolactone and oral contraceptives have become more acceptable first-line choices, and earlier use of isotretinoin has been proposed.

The evolving discoveries in atopic dermatitis (AD) shed light on disease pathogenesis and allow better management of patients. Dupiluamab was the first targeted agent approved for AD, proving for the first time AD can be treated with a single cytokine antagonism. Nevertheless, because not all patients respond to dupilumab and AD has a heterogeneous phenotype, more treatment options are much needed. This article reviews recent and exciting developments in AD, because ongoing or pipeline clinical trials for AD will ultimately expand and redefine a novel treatment paradigm for this common disease.

The treatment of refractory autoimmune blistering diseases (AIBDs) has always been a challenge. Because randomized controlled trials are lacking, treatment has been based on analysis of anecdotal data. The last 2 decades has seen the use of rituximab become a conventional treatment in the therapeutic armamentarium of AIBDs, leading to its Food and Drug Administration indication for pemphigus vulgaris in 2018. We review the current updated data on the use of rituximab including dosing, protocols, and its role in the algorithm of AIBDs. In addition, we discuss several promising novel emerging therapeutic agents for AIBDs.

The discoveries of new genes underlying genetic skin diseases have occurred at a rapid pace, supported by advances in DNA sequencing technologies. These discoveries have translated to an improved understanding of disease mechanisms at a molecular level and identified new therapeutic options based on molecular targets. This article highlights just a few of these recent discoveries for a diverse group of skin diseases, including tuberous sclerosis complex, ichthyoses, overgrowth syndromes, interferonopathies, and basal cell nevus syndrome, and how this has translated into novel targeted therapies and improved patient care.

DERMATOLOGIC CLINICS

THE CLINICS ARE AVAILABLE ONLINE!
Access your subscription at:
www.theclinics.com

Preface
Therapeutic Hotline: The Latest and Greatest in Dermatology

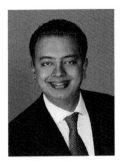

Seemal R. Desai, MD, FAAD
Editor

Dermatology is fortunate to be a specialty that encompasses a distinct and wide array of therapies; new chemical entities, reformulation of past stalwart treatments, and exciting options for rare and chronic skin diseases are on the horizon. In this issue of *Dermatologic Clinics*, I have had the privilege of creating a tour de force of the leaders in our specialty. These leaders discuss the newest and greatest updates in a variety of areas within dermatology.

Many of our readers may have attended the spectacular "Therapeutic Hotline" Symposium at the annual American Academy of Dermatology meeting. This issue of *Dermatologic Clinics* was inspired by many of those great lectures. The result is a true cornucopia spanning so many different aspects of adult and pediatric dermatology. We begin our journey with an in-depth view of "What's New in Psoriasis" and then continue with over 10 other exciting and enticing articles.

The focus of our articles is to provide you, our readers, with the most up-to-date treatment options and highlights on new therapies. This publication is not designed to be a disease state review, but rather, to allow the practicing clinician

to have quick, easy, clinically relevant access and pearls to the newest treatment options available and being studied.

I would like to thank all of the authors for their time and expertise in putting this very special issue together. In addition, my special thanks to Bruce Thiers, MD for the invitation to serve as Guest Editor, and to the team at Elsevier, in particular, Jessica McCool and Sara Watkins, for their tireless diligence. It has been a pleasure to serve as Guest Editor, and I hope you will enjoy this very special issue of *Dermatologic Clinics*.

Seemal R. Desai, MD, FAAD
Innovative Dermatology
PA, USA

Department of Dermatology
The University of Texas Southwestern Medical
Center
5425 West Spring Creek Parkway
Suite 265
Plano, TX 75024, USA

E-mail address:
seemald@yahoo.com

Dermatol Clin 37 (2019) ix
https://doi.org/10.1016/j.det.2019.01.001
0733-8635/19/© 2019 Published by Elsevier Inc.

derm.theclinics.com

What's New in Psoriasis

Stephanie von Csiky-Sessoms, Mark Lebwohl, MD*

KEYWORDS

- Psoriasis • Treatment • Interleukin-23 • Interleukin-17 • TNF-α • Biologic

KEY POINTS

- Psoriasis is a T-cell–mediated disease in which inflammatory cytokines, such as interleukin-17 (IL-17), IL-23, and tumor necrosis factor-α, play key roles in pathogenesis.
- Various biologics have been developed that target the inflammatory pathways involved in development of psoriatic disease.
- The efficacy and safety of the different treatment options have been extensively studied in the last few years in large controlled trials.

Psoriasis is a chronic, inflammatory skin disease characterized by the formation of sharply demarcated, scaly, erythematous plaques. Research over the last few decades has revealed the pathogenesis of psoriasis to be primarily an autoimmune, T-cell–mediated disease with cytokines interleukin-23 (IL-23), IL-17, and tumor necrosis factor-α (TNF-α) playing major roles in a dysregulated inflammatory response leading to the development of psoriatic lesions and associated comorbid conditions (**Fig. 1**).[1] The presentation of psoriasis varies widely among patients and is associated with a variety of comorbid conditions, including cardiometabolic disease, stroke, metabolic syndrome (obesity, hypertension, dyslipidemia, and diabetes), chronic kidney disease, gastrointestinal disease, arthritis, mood disorders, and malignancy.[1] As the understanding of the disease has deepened, more treatment options have been developed and studied, allowing one to prescribe treatments based on comorbidities.[2,3]

Research has shown that T-helper 17 (Th17) lymphocytes, a specific subset of Th1 lymphocytes, play a central role in the pathogenesis of psoriasis. These T-helper cells express proinflammatory IL-17, which upregulates the inflammation seen in psoriasis and other inflammatory disorders. IL-23, a cytokine produced by myeloid cells, expands Th17 cells and acts as a survival factor for these T-helper cells. The Th17 cells themselves release proinflammatory cytokines, such as IL-17A, IL-17F, and IL-22, which activate a cascade of cytokines and cellular mediators like IL-1, IL-6, TNF-α, and nitric oxide synthase 2 resulting in thickening of the epidermis with clustering of CD8+ T cells and neutrophils, and keratinocyte proliferation, a markedly reduced granular layer, dilation of blood vessels in the papillary dermis with inflammatory clusters containing T cells and dendritic cells, all hallmarks of psoriatic disease.[4] IL-23 is also directly proinflammatory and itself acts as a mediator of hyperproliferation and dysregulation of cutaneous cells. TNF-α, like IL-23, is a key proinflammatory cytokine that facilitates the release of other inflammatory mediators.[4] The multiplicity of therapeutic targets has resulted in the development of multiple monoclonal antibodies targeting these key mediators of the inflammatory cascade involved in the development of psoriasis (**Table 1**). With the publication of several large

Disclosure Statement: M. Lebwohl is an employee of Mount Sinai, which receives research funds from Abbvie, Amgen, Boehringer Ingelheim, Celgene, Eli Lilly, Janssen, Johnson & Johnson, Kadmon, MedImmune, AstraZeneca, Novartis, Pfizer, and ViDac, and is also a consultant for Allergan, Leopharma, and Promius. S. von Csiky-Sessoms has no conflicts of interest.
The Kimberly and Eric J. Waldman Department of Dermatology, Icahn School of Medicine at Mount Sinai, 5 East 98th Street, 5th Floor, New York, NY 10029, USA
* Corresponding author.
E-mail address: Lebwohl@aol.com

Dermatol Clin 37 (2019) 129–136
https://doi.org/10.1016/j.det.2018.11.001

derm.theclinics.com

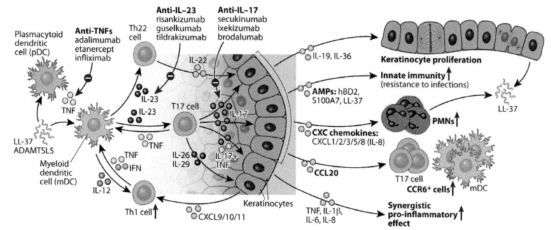

Fig. 1. IL-23/T17–mediated effects on epidermal keratinocytes in psoriatic skin. Schematic shows the broad downstream effects of increased IL-23 and IL-17 signaling on various immune cell population and keratinocyte biology. Regulated by IL-23, the primary effects of IL-17 on keratinocytes include indirect induction of epidermal hyperplasia through IL-19 and IL-36, upregulation of the innate immune response and Antimicrobial peptides (eg, hBD2, S100A7, and LL-37), epidermal recruitment of leukocyte subsets (eg, neutrophils and mDCs) through increased production of keratinocyte-derived chemokines, and transcription of multiple proinflammatory genes (eg, IL-1b, IL-6, and IL-8) that act synergistically with TNF to sustain the inflammatory events in psoriatic skin. (*From* Hawkes JE, Chan TC, Krueger JG. Psoriasis pathogenesis and the development of novel targeted immune therapies. J Allergy Clin Immunol 2017;140:648; with permission.)

randomized controlled clinical trials with these novel agents, the need to assess response with objective criteria has highlighted the key role of physician and patient disease scoring systems to assess both severity of disease and treatment outcome (**Table 2**).

INTERLEUKIN-23–TARGETED THERAPIES

IL-23 is a heterodimeric cytokine composed of a cytokine p19 subunit and a soluble alpha receptor p40 subunit, which is also found in IL-12. IL-23 binds to a receptor complex, which comprises the IL-23 receptor (IL-23R) and the IL-12 receptor β1.[5] Because IL-23 has been shown to play a major role in the pathogenesis of Th17-mediated autoimmunity and formation of plaque psoriasis lesions, this cytokine has been targeted by multiple medications (see **Table 1**).

The reSURFACE trials were a 3-part, double-blind, randomized controlled study comparing *tildrakizumab*, which targets the IL-23 p19 subunit, placebo, and etanercept. The study found that 66% in the 200-mg group and 61% in the 100-mg group achieved Psoriasis Area and Severity Index (PASI) 75, compared with 6% in the placebo group and 48% in the etanercept group. Fifty-nine percent in the 200-mg group, and 55% in the 100-mg group achieved a PGA (Physician's Global Assessment) response with a score of 0 or 1 (clear or almost clear), compared

with 4% in the placebo group and 48% in the etanercept group.[6] The adverse events were comparable and low in all of the groups, suggesting that tildrakizumab is both effective and well tolerated. Another study showed that up to 64 weeks of tildrakizumab treatment was well tolerated and had low rates of serious adverse events, discontinuations due to adverse events, or adverse events of clinical interest.[7] Response was maintained with 84%, 52%, and 22% of patients treated with the 100-mg dose achieving PASI 75, 90, and 100, respectively. These data indicate that tildrakizumab may be safe and tolerable in patients for long-term treatment of psoriasis as well. On July 27, 2018, an Almirall press release stated that they received a positive opinion from the European Medicines Agency for tildrakizumab for the treatment of patients with moderate to severe chronic plaque psoriasis.[8]

VOYAGE 1 and VOYAGE 2 were 2 phase 3 clinical trials designed to assess the efficacy of *guselkumab*, a monoclonal antibody targeting IL-23 p19, in the treatment of from moderate to severe plaque-type psoriasis. In both trials, guselkumab was found to be more effective in the treatment of moderate to severe plaque-type psoriasis when compared with both placebo and adalimumab with a greater proportion of patients achieving PASI 75, PASI 90, and PASI 100 throughout 48 weeks of treatment.[9–12] Additional studies showed that guselkumab can be used

Table 1
Biologics and other novel agents approved or under clinical investigation for treatment of psoriasis in the United States

Molecule	Name (US)	Molecular Target	FDA Status	Administration
Adalimumab	Humira Amjevita (BioS) Cyltezo (BioS)	TNF-α	Approved	SC
Certolizumab	Cimzia	TNF-α	Approved	SC
Etanercept	Enbrel Erelzi (BioS)	TNF-α	Approved	SC
Infliximab	Remicade Inflectra (BioS) Ixifi (BioS) Renflexis (BioS)	TNF-α	Approved	IV
Ixekizumab	TALTZ	IL-17A	Approved[a]	SC
Secukinumab	COSENTYX	IL-17A	Approved	SC
Brodalumab	SILIQ	IL-17R	Approved	SC
Bimekizumab	—	IL-17A/F	Phase 3	SC
Ustekinumab	STELARA	IL-12, IL23 p40	Approved	SC/IV
Guselkumab	TREMFYA	IL-23 p19	Approved	SC
Risankizumab	—	IL-23 p19	Filed[b]	SC
Tildrakizumab	ILUMYA	IL-23 p19	Approved	SC
Mirikizumab	—	IL-23 p19	Phase 3	SC/IV
Apremilast	Otezla	PDE4	Approved	Oral
Tofacitinib	HELJANZ	JAK	Approved for psoriatic arthritis	Oral

Abbreviations: BioS, biosimilar, listed only if FDA approved; IV, intravenous; SC, subcutaneous.
[a] Label updated on May 22, 2018 to include data in psoriasis involving the genital area.
[b] Submitted to the FDA on April 25, 2018, see: https://news.abbvie.com/alert-topics/immunology/abbvie-submits-biologics-license-application-to-us-fda-for-investigational-treatment-risankizumab-for-moderate-to-severe-plaque-psoriasis.htm.

effectively as maintenance therapy in patients with moderate to severe plaque-type psoriasis, because a better persistence of response was seen in patients treated with a maintenance dose from week 28 to 48, compared with patients in whom guselkumab was withdrawn.[12] A recently published secondary analysis of the 2 VOYAGE trials focused on the efficacy of guselkumab in the treatment of psoriasis in specific body regions (scalp, palms, and/or soles, and fingernails).[11] The analysis found a greater portion of guselkumab treated patients achieved clearance of scalp, palms and soles when compared to adulimumab treated patients. However, the responses were comparable for fingernail psoriasis after six months of treatment with guselkumab or adalimumab.[11] Thus, guselkumab may be a good option for the treatment of patients suffering from psoriasis in difficult-to-treat areas such as the scalp.

Although the mean age of onset of psoriasis has been found to be around 28 years, 10% of patients experience early onset before 10 years of age and 35% of patients experience early onset before 20 years of age.[13] There have been very few pediatric clinical trials done to assess the effectiveness of biologic agents for the treatment of psoriasis. *Ustekinumab* targets the p40 subunit shared by IL-12 and IL-23. It has been shown to be safe and effective for the treatment of moderate to severe plaque psoriasis in adults. The CADMUS study was a randomized, double-blind, placebo-controlled study enrolling patients between the ages of 12 and 17 with moderate to severe plaque psoriasis. The study found that patients in both the standard dose and the half-standard dose groups experienced a significant clinical improvement with more than half of patients in both groups achieving PASI 90 at 12 weeks of treatment.[14] Furthermore, there were no unexpected adverse effects reported during the study. The findings of the CADMUS study suggest that ustekinumab could be an effective treatment option for adolescent patients suffering from moderate to severe plaque psoriasis. However, several adult studies

Table 2
Psoriasis assessment tools

Scoring System	Patient or Provider Assessed	Description and Interpretation
PASI (Psoriasis Area and Severity Index)	Provider	Measure of the average redness, thickness, and scaliness of lesions (each graded on a 0–4 scale), weighted by the area of involvement
PASI 75 (Psoriasis area and Severity Index 75)	Provider	75% improvement in PASI score
PASI 90 (Psoriasis Area and Severity Index 90)	Provider	90% improvement in PASI score
PASI 100 (Psoriasis Area and Severity Index 100)	Provider	100% improvement in PASI score
sPGA (Static Physician Global Assessment)	Provider	Physicians impression of disease Severe: marked plaque elevation, scaling, and/or erythema Moderate to severe: Marked plaque elevation, scaling, and/or erythema Moderate: Moderate plaque elevation, scaling, and/or erythema Mild to moderate: Intermediate between moderate and mild Mild: Slight plaque elevation, scaling, and/or erythema Almost clear: Intermediate between mild and clear Clear: No signs of psoriasis
BSA (body surface area)	Provider	Percent of body covered by lesions
PSI (Psoriasis Symptom Inventory)	Patient	Range, 0–32, with higher scores indicating more severe disease
DLQI (Dermatology Life Quality Index)	Patient	0–1, no effect at all on patient's life 2–5, small effect on patient's life 6–10, moderate effect on patient's life 11–20, very large effect on patient's life 21–30, extremely large effect on patient's life

have shown inferiority of ustekinumab in head-to-head comparisons with other products, including ixekizumab (IXORA-S),[15,16] secukinumab (CLEAR),[17] risankizumab (UltIMMa-1 and UltIMMa-2),[18] and brodalumab (AMAGINE-2 and AMAGINE-3).[19]

Risankizumab is a humanized immunoglobulin G1 monoclonal antibody targeting IL-23 p19. The pivotal phase 3 trials (UltIMMa-1 and UltIMMa-2), which support the recent filing for Food and Drug Administration (FDA) approval, are being published. These trials tested the efficacy in moderate to severe chronic plaque psoriasis of 150 mg risankizumab subcutaneously versus either placebo or 2 different doses (45 or 90 mg) of ustekinumab.[18] After 16 weeks of therapy, in the UltIMMa-1 trial, PASI 90 was achieved by 75.3% of patients receiving risankizumab versus 42.0% for ustekinumab-treated patients (adjusted different 33.5%, range 22.7%–44.3%). In UltIMMa-1, Static Physician Global Assessment (sPGA) values of 0 or 1 were achieved by

87.8% of patients receiving risankizumab versus 63.0% for ustekinumab-treated patients (adjusted different 25.1%, range 15.2%–35.0%). Essentially similar responses were observed in the UtIIMMa-2 trial.

INTERLEUKIN-17–TARGETED THERAPIES

Th17 cells are a subset of T cells that express IL-17, are expanded in the presence of IL-23, and have been shown to play a key role in psoriasis, mostly based on their capability to produce IL-17.[20] IL-17 and TNF-α are synergistic in their capability of activating key inflammatory responses in psoriasis.

Brodalumab is a fully human monoclonal antibody targeting the IL-17 receptor A. It been shown to be effective in the treatment of plaque psoriasis.[19,21] The AMAGINE-2 and AMAGINE-3 clinical trials were double-blind, placebo- and ustekinumab-controlled phase 3 clinical trials designed to assess the efficacy and safety of brodalumab. These trials demonstrated that brodalumab treatment resulted in significant clinical improvement in patients with moderate to severe psoriasis.[19] Both studies were designed with a 12-week induction followed by a 40-week maintenance phase. Brodalumab was found to have higher efficacy in both the AMAGINE-2 and AMAGINE-3 trials with respect to PASI and sPGA scores. Brodalumab treatment resulted in superior PASI 75, 90, and 100 results (85.7%, 69.5%, and 40.5% of patients, respectively) when compared with ustekinumab (69.7%, 47.3%, and 20.1%, respectively, all P<.001). Furthermore, more Brodalumab patients achieved sPGA (0/1) at week 12 than ustekinumab patients (79.1% vs 59.1%, P<.001).[21] It is also of note that the efficacy of brodalumab in biologic-experienced patients was 3 times higher than the efficacy of ustekinumab in biologic-experienced patients for PASI 100 (32% vs 11.3%). Efficacy rates may differ between patients who are biologic-naive versus biologic-experienced patients who have failed or discontinued a biologic medication in the past.[19] Papp and colleagues[22] used the AMAGINE-2 and AMAGINE-3 study data to analyze the impact of previous biologic use of on the efficacy and safety of both brodalumab and ustekinumab. The analysis showed brodalumab demonstrated similar efficacy (P = .31, .32, and 0.64 for PASI 75, 90, and 100, respectively) in biologic-naive and biologic-experienced patients, demonstrating that prior biologic exposure does not affect the disease outcomes in patients treated with brodalumab. There was also a substantial and rapid improvement in lesional symptoms (itch, assessed by PSI [Psoriasis Symptom Inventory]) in patients treated with brodalumab versus both placebo and ustekinumab, especially in patients with moderate to very severe itch scores (>1) and in those who achieved complete clearance response.[23]

Ixekizumab is a monoclonal antibody that selectively binds IL-17A and has shown activity in moderate and severe psoriasis.[24–27] IL-17 is thought to be central in the pathogenesis of psoriatic arthritis, a chronic inflammatory arthritis associated with psoriasis. IL-17 activates immune cells resulting in production of inflammatory cytokines and chemokines resulting in the recruitment of neutrophils and monocytes, and the release of metalloproteases, which destroy cartilage and activate receptor activator of nuclear factor κ-B ligand, which destroys bone resulting in joint degeneration and arthritis.[28] A recent study (SPIRIT-P1), a double-blind placebo- and adalimumab-controlled 3-year phase 3 trial, explored the efficacy of ixekizumab in the treatment of psoriatic arthritis specifically in biologic-naive patients.[29]

The study found that 80 mg ixekizumab given every 2 weeks or every 4 weeks following a starting dose of 160 mg at week 0 significantly improved psoriatic arthritis symptoms such as enthesitis and dactylitis, and also significantly improved patient-reported physical functioning. Radiographic findings demonstrated that ixekizumab inhibited radiographic progression of joint destruction when compared with placebo.[29] Another study focused on psoriatic arthritis showed that ixekizumab was essentially similar to adalimumab in reducing disease activity, functional disabilities, and progression of structural damage.[30] The IXORA-P study assessed the efficacy of a continuous biweekly 80-mg dose of ixekizumab over 52 weeks of treatment, which is a treatment time substantially longer than the original 12 weeks of the labeling studies.[31] This study showed the superiority of dosing ixekizumab every 2 weeks over every 4 weeks, with 60% of patients showing a PASI 100 response at 52 weeks versus 49% in the every 4 weeks dosing. However, this every 2 week dosing was associated with a significant increase in injection site reactions compared with the every 4 week dosing, and a significant increase in serious infections, oral candidiasis, and hypersensitivity reactions over placebo. Recent studies have shown that ixekizumab is highly effective for genital psoriasis regardless of the body surface area (BSA), with significant improvements shown in both itch and sexual function, with 7/10 patients achieving clear or almost clear genital skin at week 12 of treatment, and with 8/10 treated patients no longer or rarely limited by the impact of genital psoriasis on sexual activity at week 12.[32]

Secukinumab is another biologic therapy that selectively targets IL-17A shown to have significant efficacy in the treatment of moderate to severe psoriasis and psoriatic arthritis.[33,34] The SCULPTURE extension study examined the efficacy and safety of secukizumab use through 5 consecutive years.[35] The study found persistence of response to secukinumab over the 5-year period, with more than three-fourths of subjects completing 5 years of treatment.[35] Furthermore, secukinumab improved psoriasis on average by 90% over 5 years, with mean improvement of 91.1% in mean absolute PASI from baseline to year 1, and of 90.1% from baseline to year 5. Similarly, there were sustained improvements in mean absolute BSA from baseline to year 1 of 92.2% and to year 5, of 92.2% and 91.8%, respectively. There was also no increase in yearly adverse effect rates from year 1 to year 5, and the safety profile remained favorable throughout 5 years of treatment.[35] Quality-of-life indicators collected in the

CLEAR study[17] have shown superiority of secukinumab over ustekinumab for complete pain relief, and for faster complete relief of itching and scaling.[36]

Bimekizumab is a novel monoclonal antibody with neutralizing properties against both IL-17A and IL-17F.[37] Phase 2 results have been presented for moderate to severe plaque psoriasis (BE ABLE) and for psoriatic arthritis (BE ACTIVE). Bimekizumab achieved a 79% PASI 90 response rate and a 62% PASI 100 response rate, and 46% of patients experience a 50% improvement in joint symptoms in the psoriatic arthritis study.[38]

TUMOR NECROSIS FACTOR–TARGETED THERAPIES

A recent study with *Adalimumab* in patients with moderate to severe fingernails psoriasis and at least 5% BSA involvement has shown substantial clinical benefits and has resulted in the addition of this indication to the drug label.[39] A modified Nail Psoriasis Severity Index (mNAPSI) was used in the study, which showed an mNAPSI 75 response rate in 46.6% of treated patient at week 26 versus 3.4% for placebo.

Certolizumab pegol is a novel, Fc-free, PEGylated, monoclonal antibody targeting TNF, which at 16 weeks of therapy showed PASI 90 response rates of 39.8% (200 mg every 2 weeks) and 49.1% (400 mg every 2 weeks) with no unexpected side effects (CIMPACT).[40] Two additional large trials (CIMPASI-1 and CIMPASI-2) examined the effects of 48 weeks of therapy and showed PASI 75 response rates of 83.6% (400 mg every 2 weeks) and 70.7% (200 mg every 2 weeks) with PASI 90 response rates of 61.6% (400 mg every 2 weeks) and 50.0% (200 mg every 2 weeks).[41]

Etanercept is another TNF-targeted psoriasis therapy. The largest and longest pediatric study with biologics in psoriasis reported to date looked at the efficacy and safety of etanercept in children and adolescents with plaque psoriasis.[42] The percentages of patients achieving PASI 75 and PASI 90 responses from baseline remained relatively constant at approximately 60% to 70% and 30% to 40%, respectively, at week 96 through week 264. Similarly, the percentage of patients who achieved sPGA status of clear/almost clear (score 0/1) remained relatively constant at approximately 40% to 50% from week 96 through week 264.[42] Furthermore, no new safety concerns were uncovered during the course of the study, which suggests that the efficacy and safety previously reported in adult populations may be generalizable to pediatric populations.

REFERENCES

1. Hawkes JE, Chan TC, Krueger JG. Psoriasis pathogenesis and the development of novel targeted immune therapies. J Allergy Clin Immunol 2017; 140(3):645–53.
2. Kaushik SB, Lebwohl MG. CME part I psoriasis: which therapy for which patient psoriasis comorbidities and preferred systemic agents. J Am Acad Dermatol 2018. https://doi.org/10.1016/j.jaad.2018.06.057.
3. Kaushik SB, Lebwohl MG. CME part II psoriasis: which therapy for which patient focus on special populations and chronic infections. J Am Acad Dermatol 2018. https://doi.org/10.1016/j.jaad.2018.06.056.
4. Boehncke WH. Etiology and pathogenesis of psoriasis. Rheum Dis Clin North Am 2015;41(4):665–75.
5. Bloch Y, Bouchareychas L, Merceron R, et al. Structural activation of pro-inflammatory human cytokine IL-23 by cognate IL-23 receptor enables recruitment of the shared receptor IL-12rbeta1. Immunity 2018; 48(1):45–58.e6.
6. Reich K, Papp KA, Blauvelt A, et al. Tildrakizumab versus placebo or etanercept for chronic plaque psoriasis (reSURFACE 1 and reSURFACE 2): results from two randomised controlled, phase 3 trials. Lancet 2017;390(10091):276–88.
7. Blauvelt A, Reich K, Papp KA, et al. Safety of tildrakizumab for moderate-to-severe plaque psoriasis: pooled analysis of three randomized controlled trials. Br J Dermatol 2018. https://doi.org/10.1111/bjd.16724.
8. Almirall. Almirall receives positive CHMP opinion for new anti-IL23 tildrakizumab for the treatment of patients with moderate-to-severe chronic plaque psoriasis. Secondary Almirall receives positive CHMP opinion for new anti-IL23 tildrakizumab for the treatment of patients with moderate-to-severe chronic plaque psoriasis 2018. Available at: https://www.almirall.com/en/media/press-releases/media-detail-new?title=almirall-receives-positive-chmp-opinion-for-new-anti-il23-tildrakizumab-for-the-treatment-of-patients-with-moderate-to-severe-chronic-plaque-psoriasis&articleId=3229603. Accessed October 2, 2018.
9. Blauvelt A, Papp KA, Griffiths CEM, et al. Efficacy and safety of guselkumab, an anti-interleukin-23 monoclonal antibody, compared with adalimumab for the continuous treatment of patients with moderate to severe psoriasis: results from the phase III, double-blinded, placebo- and active comparator-controlled VOYAGE 1 trial. J Am Acad Dermatol 2017;76(3):405–17.
10. Gordon KB, Blauvelt A, Foley P, et al. Efficacy of guselkumab in subpopulations of patients with moderate-to-severe plaque psoriasis: a pooled

analysis of the phase III VOYAGE 1 and VOYAGE 2 studies. Br J Dermatol 2018;178(1):132–9.

11. Foley P, Gordon K, Griffiths CEM, et al. Efficacy of guselkumab compared with adalimumab and placebo for psoriasis in specific body regions: a secondary analysis of 2 randomized clinical trials. JAMA Dermatol 2018;154(6):676–83.

12. Reich K, Armstrong AW, Foley P, et al. Efficacy and safety of guselkumab, an anti-interleukin-23 monoclonal antibody, compared with adalimumab for the treatment of patients with moderate to severe psoriasis with randomized withdrawal and retreatment: Results from the phase III, double-blind, placebo- and active comparator-controlled VOYAGE 2 trial. J Am Acad Dermatol 2017; 76(3):418–31.

13. Farber EM, Nall ML. The natural history of psoriasis in 5,600 patients. Dermatologica 1974;148(1):1–18.

14. Landells I, Marano C, Hsu MC, et al. Ustekinumab in adolescent patients age 12 to 17 years with moderate-to-severe plaque psoriasis: results of the randomized phase 3 CADMUS study. J Am Acad Dermatol 2015;73(4):594–603.

15. Reich K, Pinter A, Lacour JP, et al. Comparison of ixekizumab with ustekinumab in moderate-to-severe psoriasis: 24-week results from IXORA-S, a phase III study. Br J Dermatol 2017;177(4):1014–23.

16. Paul C, Griffiths CEM, van de Kerkhof PCM, et al. Ixekizumab provides superior efficacy compared to ustekinumab over 52-weeks of treatment: results from IXORA-S, a phase 3 study. J Am Acad Dermatol 2018. https://doi.org/10.1016/j.jaad.2018.06.039.

17. Blauvelt A, Reich K, Tsai TF, et al. Secukinumab is superior to ustekinumab in clearing skin of subjects with moderate-to-severe plaque psoriasis up to 1 year: results from the CLEAR study. J Am Acad Dermatol 2017;76(1):60–9.e9.

18. Gordon KB, Strober B, Lebwohl M, et al. Efficacy and safety of risankizumab in moderate-to-severe plaque psoriasis (UltIMMa-1 and UltIMMa-2): results from two double-blind, randomised, placebo-controlled and ustekinumab-controlled phase 3 trials. Lancet 2018. https://doi.org/10.1016/S0140-6736(18)31713-6.

19. Lebwohl M, Strober B, Menter A, et al. Phase 3 studies comparing brodalumab with ustekinumab in psoriasis. N Engl J Med 2015;373(14): 1318–28.

20. Martin DA, Towne JE, Kricorian G, et al. The emerging role of IL-17 in the pathogenesis of psoriasis: preclinical and clinical findings. J Invest Dermatol 2013;133(1):17–26.

21. Papp KA, Reich K, Paul C, et al. A prospective phase III, randomized, double-blind, placebo-controlled study of brodalumab in patients with moderate-to-severe plaque psoriasis. Br J Dermatol 2016;175(2):273–86.

22. Papp KA, Gordon KB, Langley RG, et al. Impact of previous biologic use on the efficacy and safety of brodalumab and ustekinumab in patients with moderate-to-severe plaque psoriasis: integrated analysis of the randomized controlled trials AMAGINE-2 and AMAGINE-3. Br J Dermatol 2018. https://doi.org/10.1111/bjd.16464.

23. Gottlieb AB, Gordon K, Hsu S, et al. Improvement in itch and other psoriasis symptoms with brodalumab in phase 3 randomized controlled trials. J Eur Acad Dermatol Venereol 2018;32(8):1305–13.

24. Leonardi C, Matheson R, Zachariae C, et al. Anti–interleukin-17 monoclonal antibody ixekizumab in chronic plaque psoriasis. N Engl J Med 2012; 366(13):1190–9.

25. Gordon KB, Blauvelt A, Papp KA, et al. Phase 3 trials of ixekizumab in moderate-to-severe plaque psoriasis. N Engl J Med 2016;375(4):345–56.

26. Gordon KB, Leonardi CL, Lebwohl M, et al. A 52-week, open-label study of the efficacy and safety of ixekizumab, an anti-interleukin-17A monoclonal antibody, in patients with chronic plaque psoriasis. J Am Acad Dermatol 2014;71(6):1176–82.

27. van der Heijde D, Gladman DD, Kishimoto M, et al. Efficacy and safety of ixekizumab in patients with active psoriatic arthritis: 52-week results from a phase III study (SPIRIT-P1). J Rheumatol 2018;45(3):367–77.

28. Raychaudhuri SP. Role of IL-17 in psoriasis and psoriatic arthritis. Clin Rev Allergy Immunol 2013;44(2): 183–93.

29. Mease PJ, van der Heijde D, Ritchlin CT, et al. Ixekizumab, an interleukin-17A specific monoclonal antibody, for the treatment of biologic-naive patients with active psoriatic arthritis: results from the 24-week randomised, double-blind, placebo-controlled and active (adalimumab)-controlled period of the phase III trial SPIRIT-P1. Ann Rheum Dis 2017;76(1):79–87.

30. Warren RB, Brnabic A, Saure D, et al. Matching-adjusted indirect comparison of efficacy in patients with moderate-to-severe plaque psoriasis treated with ixekizumab vs. secukinumab. Br J Dermatol 2018;178(5):1064–71.

31. Langley RG, Papp K, Gooderham M, et al. Efficacy and safety of continuous every-2-week dosing of ixekizumab over 52 weeks in patients with moderate-to-severe plaque psoriasis in a randomized phase III trial (IXORA-P). Br J Dermatol 2018;178(6): 1315–23.

32. Ryan C, Menter A, Guenther L, et al. Efficacy and safety of ixekizumab in a randomized, double-blinded, placebo-controlled, phase 3B clinical trial in patients with moderate-to-severe genital psoriasis. J Sex Med 2018;15(2):S6–7.

33. Langley RG, Elewski BE, Lebwohl M, et al. Secukinumab in plaque psoriasis–results of two phase 3 trials. N Engl J Med 2014;371(4):326–38.

34. Mease PJ, McInnes IB, Kirkham B, et al. Secukinumab inhibition of interleukin-17A in patients with psoriatic arthritis. N Engl J Med 2015;373(14):1329–39.

35. Bissonnette R, Luger T, Thaçi D, et al. Secukinumab demonstrates high sustained efficacy and a favourable safety profile in patients with moderate-to-severe psoriasis through 5 years of treatment (SCULPTURE Extension Study). J Eur Acad Dermatol Venereol 2018. https://doi.org/10.1111/jdv.14878.

36. Puig L, Augustin M, Blauvelt A, et al. Effect of secukinumab on quality of life and psoriasis-related symptoms: a comparative analysis versus ustekinumab from the CLEAR 52-week study. J Am Acad Dermatol 2018;78(4):741–8.

37. Glatt S, Baeten D, Baker T, et al. Dual IL-17A and IL-17F neutralisation by bimekizumab in psoriatic arthritis: evidence from preclinical experiments and a randomised placebo-controlled clinical trial that IL-17F contributes to human chronic tissue inflammation. Ann Rheum Dis 2018;77(4):523–32.

38. Papp KA, Merola JF, Gottlieb AB, et al. Dual neutralization of both interleukin 17A and interleukin 17F with bimekizumab in patients with psoriasis: Results from BE ABLE 1, a 12-week randomized, double-blinded, placebo-controlled phase 2b trial. J Am Acad Dermatol 2018;79(2):277.

39. Elewski BE, Okun MM, Papp K, et al. Adalimumab for nail psoriasis: efficacy and safety from the first 26 weeks of a phase 3, randomized, placebo-controlled trial. J Am Acad Dermatol 2018;78(1):90–9.e1.

40. Lebwohl M, Blauvelt A, Paul C, et al. Certolizumab pegol for the treatment of chronic plaque psoriasis: Results through 48 weeks of a phase 3, multicenter, randomized, double-blind, etanercept- and placebo-controlled study (CIMPACT). J Am Acad Dermatol 2018;79(2):266–76.e5.

41. Gottlieb AB, Blauvelt A, Thaçi D, et al. Certolizumab pegol for the treatment of chronic plaque psoriasis: results through 48 weeks from 2 phase 3, multicenter, randomized, double-blinded, placebo-controlled studies (CIMPASI-1 and CIMPASI-2). J Am Acad Dermatol 2018;79(2):302–14.e6.

42. Paller AS, Siegfried EC, Pariser DM, et al. Long-term safety and efficacy of etanercept in children and adolescents with plaque psoriasis. J Am Acad Dermatol 2016;74(2):280–7.e1-3.

What's New in Hair Loss

Leopoldo Duailibe Nogueira Santos, MD[a,b,c,d], Jerry Shapiro, MD, FRCP[b],*

KEYWORDS

- Androgenetic alopecia • Frontal fibrosing alopecia • Alopecia areata • Platelet-rich plasma
- Isotretinoin • Acitretin • Retinoid • Janus kinase inhibitors

KEY POINTS

- The number of frontal fibrosing alopecia patients has dramatically increased over the past years.
- New drugs, such as retinoids, are urged to halt the hair loss progression.
- Alopecia areata has an important impact on patient quality of life. To date, there is no Food and Drug Administration–approved treatment.
- Janus Kinase (JAK) inhibitors have shown promising results in the treatment of alopecia areata.
- The 5α-reductase side-effect profile is a concern for many patients. Platelet-rich plasma is a possible solution to fill this gap in androgenetic alopecia treatment.

INTRODUCTION

Hair loss has an important impact on patient quality of life. Therefore, many patients are seeking medical advice to stop their hair loss progression or gain more hairs.

Frontal fibrosing alopecia (FFA) is a new cicatricial alopecia (CA) first described in 1994 by Kossard.[1] Since then, the number of cases has increased exponentially. There are a lot of similarities between lichen planopilaris and FFA. Histopathologically, the perifollicular lymphocytic infiltrates are indistinguishable. Therefore, FFA is classified as an autoimmune disease and lymphocyte-mediated scarring alopecia within the lichen planopilaris group.[2–4] On the other hand, opposite of lichen planopilaris, FFA is more prevalent in women approximately in their 50s and, rarely, seen in men. Also, 5α-reductase blockers, such as finasteride and dutasteride, may help stop the hair loss progression. These findings corroborate a hormonal etiology.[2–4]

CA eliminates the hair follicle and results in scarring. CAs are considered a trichologic emergency and combination therapy is necessary.[5] In the FFA group, many dermatologists opt to start treatment using medications from the hormonal and autoimmune mechanisms combined. Not all patients, however, respond to this approach. Retinoids are a new class of drugs in the arsenal, striking against this form of alopecia.

Androgenetic alopecia (AGA) is the most prevalent form of hair loss in men, affecting approximately 50% of the patients by the time they reach 50 years of age.[6] The main Food and Drug Administration–approved AGA treatments for men are topical minoxidil and oral finasteride. Although controversial, concern about oral finasteride's sexual end fertility side effects has increased among patients.[7] Patients often seek consultations to avoid finasteride and research different treatments, even if they are told about the well-established efficacy of finasteride. Platelet-rich plasma (PRP), an

Disclosure Statement: L.D.N. Santos: no conflict of interest; J. Shapiro: Pfiizer, Aclaris, Incyte, Bioniz, Replicel Life Sciences, and Applied Biology.
[a] Santa Casa of São Paulo School of Medicine, Rua Doutor Cesário Motta Júnior 61, São Paulo, SP 01221-020, Brazil; [b] Municipal Public Servant Hospital of São Paulo, Rua Castro Alves 60, São Paulo, SP 01532-000, Brazil; [c] University of Taubaté, Av. Granadeiro Guimarães 270, Taubaté, SP 12020-130, Brazil; [d] The Ronald O. Perelman Department of Dermatology, New York University School of Medicine, 530 First Avenue, Suite 7R, New York, NY 10016, USA
* Corresponding author.
E-mail address: jerry.shapiro@nyumc.org

Dermatol Clin 37 (2019) 137–141
https://doi.org/10.1016/j.det.2018.11.002

autologous form of treatment, is a new option for such patients.

The lifetime incidence risk of alopecia areata is 2.1% in the general population. Most patients develop only a few patches and respond well to corticosteroid lotions or injections. Some patients notice hair regrowth without treatment. The treatment of alopecia universalis or alopecia totalis, however, is challenging. There is no treatment approved by the Food and Drug Administration. The translational work using the JAK inhibitors has a great potential to change this scenario.[8,9]

FRONTAL FIBROSING ALOPECIA
Isotretinoin

Recently, Rakowska and colleagues[10] published the benefit of retinoids in treating FFA. This retrospective study compared 3 treatment groups: low-dose isotretinoin (20 mg/d), low-dose acitretin (20 mg/d), and finasteride (5 mg/d). The assessment was made measuring the distance between the glabella crease and frontal hairline. Hair loss progression was halted in 76% patients using low-dose isotretinoin, 73% in the low-dose acitretin group, and 43% in the finasteride group. Although these are the only available data using retinoids in FFA, they are a breakthrough in the treatment of FFA.

The peroxisome proliferator-activated receptors (PPARs) regulate the expression of genes involved with lipid metabolism, and PPAR-γ deficiency has been associated with the lichen planopilaris. This lipid metabolism change should be the cause rather than the consequence of expression of proinflammatory pathways. PPAR-γ agonists (eg, pioglitazone) have shown some efficacy treating lichen planopilaris.[11–15]

The investigators of the FFA and retinoids study mention that the mechanism of action should be its anti-keratinization process; however, the possible mechanism of action of retinoids might be the up-regulation of PPAR-γ, because lowdose retinoic acid demonstrated activating PPAR-γ.[16] Although retinoids might be a promising treatment for FFA, the authors advocate combination treatment (topical, intralesional triamcinolone acetonide and/or systemic medications) in the beginning of the treatment plan. After stabilization of the disease, the tapering process may be initiated.

ANDROGENETIC ALOPECIA
Platelet-rich Plasma

Introduction

PRP is an autologous blood product. Hematologists coined the PRP term in the 1970s, when treating patients with thrombocytopenia. Afterward, other medical specialties have started using PRP, including sports medicine, orthopedics, plastic surgery, gynecology, and dentistry.[17]

Dermatology has increased its attention on PRP more recently. Specifically, in the fields of wound healing, cosmetic dermatology, and hair loss. PRP has been proposed as an efficacious treatment of AGA and alopecia areata, with some benefit for CAs.[18–20]

Rationale

The rationale involving PRP and hair loss is associated with its concentrated number of growth factors (GFs) that stimulate hair regrowth. PRP contains, depending on the protocol, a 1.2-fold to 9-fold increase in platelet concentration compared with complete blood cell count. Platelets contain many granules, a rich source of myriad GFs. Some GFs may be associated with increased hair regrowth. Paradoxically, other GFs may inhibit hair regrowth.[17,21] Therefore, there must be a perfect balance of GFs to promote hair regrowth.

Pathways involved are the Wnt/β-catenin signaling and activation of extracellular signal-regulated kinase and protein kinase B (Akt) signaling.[17,21] As a consequence, PRP has been proposed to increase proliferation and cell survival of dermal papilla cells and a faster telogen-anagen transition.[17,21]

Androgens attaching to androgen receptors on hair follicles may block many of these pathways, discussed previously, inhibiting the manufacture and release of GFs and, therefore, inhibiting hair regrowth. Girijala and colleagues propose an interesting idea regarding the mechanism of action citing that PRP may be a vehicle through which the complex process of growth factor production can be bypassed.[22]

Protocol

There are several methods via which PRP can be obtained Many clinical trials do not specify all the various characteristics of how PRP was obtained. To date, there is no standardized protocol. Generally, blood is drawn from a patient by venipuncture in a tube containing anticoagulant (sodium citrate or EDTA). Then, the tube is spun 1 or 2 cycles in a centrifuge. After centrifuging, there are 3 distinct layers (from top to bottom): platelet-poor plasma (PPP); buffy coat (BC), rich in platelets and white blood cells; and red blood cells. In certain protocols, a second cycle is recommended using PPP and BC. The second centrifugation results in a final product with a higher concentration of platelets—PRP. Depending on the protocol, PPP plus BC

(1 cycle) or PRP (2 cycles) can be used for hair loss treatment.[23–25]

Many metrics of PRP processing can influence the result of the final product: initial whole blood volume, number of spins, spin rate, spin time, gravitational force of the centrifuge, and centrifuge machine. As a result, all these different metrics make a comparison among clinical trials challenging, not to mention that not all data are listed in published literature. For example, only 32% of literature shows initial and final platelet counts.[23]

Activation is another controversial topic. Some investigators claim that activating PRP with thrombin, calcium chloride, or calcium gluconate releases more GFs and, therefore, promotes more hair regrowth. On the other hand, more inhibitory GFs are released, causing the opposite effect.[23,25]

Results

In the last five years the number of published studies about PRP and hair loss has increased. On the other hand, only a few are well designed and most of them analyze different parameters, thus comparing them all turns out to be difficult.

Alves and Grimalt[26] found no difference in hair count after PRP treatment; however, there were increases in terminal hairs and total hair density. Cervelli and colleagues[27] and Gentile and colleagues[28] also had positive results in hair density, terminal hairs and hair count.

Mapar and colleagues[29] were not fortunate with their results and there was no improvement in terminal hair count and vellus hair count. Similarly, Puig and colleagues[30] did not see any increase in hair mass index. The main criticism of these 2 trials is the number of injection sessions (1 and 2, respectively). Plus, Puig and colleagues[30] did not activate PRP, possibly lowering the number of GFs released.

Recently, Ayatollahi and colleagues[31] published a case series of PRP treatment and demonstrated no benefit using a single-spin protocol. The short-term 3-month follow-up plus many induced telogen effluvium might raise a question if a longer follow-up would show better results. Hausauer and Jones[32] using a different single-spin kit compared 2 injection protocols: 3 monthly sessions with a booster 3 months later (total 4 treatments; group 1) versus 1 session every 3 months (total 2 treatments; group 2). Both groups reproduced positive results at 6 months; however, if the follow-up period had been longer, the results could have been different due to a high rate of induced telogen effluvium and a short follow-up period of 3 month and was more pronounced at 6-month assessment (hair count improvement at 6 months, 29.6% × 7.2%, respectively).[32]

Based on the literature, discussed previously, and the authors' experience, the following protocol is proposed for better and faster results. If there is no improvement after 2 months' to 4 months' follow-up, PRP might not work for a specific patient. Always bear in mind that combination therapy is important to achieve real-world outcomes.[18]

Proposed protocol
- Initial treatment: monthly, 6 months
- Maintenance: every 3 months

ALOPECIA AREATA
Janus Kinase Inhibitors

Introduction
Genome-wide association studies demonstrated that autoimmune diseases (alopecia areata, rheumatoid arthritis, and type 1 diabetes mellitus) share similar pathological changes within the Janus Kinase and Signal Transducer and Activator of Transcription (JAK-STAT) signaling. Further mouse models studies proved the rationale of this pathogenic signaling in alopecia areata. Since then, JAK inhibitors have gained much attention in the hair field.[33,34]

The pathway
Many extracellular cytokines and other molecules generate gene expression using the JAK-STAT signaling pathway. There are 4 JAKs and 7 STATs making possible combinations. Dysregulated activation of this pathway or a response to JAK inhibitors has been associated with several autoimmune diseases (psoriasis, vitiligo, atopic dermatitis, alopecia areata, rheumatoid arthritis, and so forth).[35,36]

Interleukin 15 (IL-15) and interferon gamma (IFN-γ) have shown important roles in alopecia areata. Also, these 2 cytokines were associated with JAK signaling, corroborating the hypothesis that the JAK-STAT pathways are involved in alopecia areata.[35,36]

Oral
The studied JAK inhibitors for alopecia areata are tofacitinib (mostly inhibiting JAK1 and JAK3), ruxolitinib (selective for JAK1 and JAK2), and to a lesser extent baricitinib (selective for JAK1 and JAK2).[37,38]

Many patients responded dramatically, with response rates of approximately 75% in many studies. A study with 12 patients showed similar response rates between patchy alopecia and alopecia totalis/universalis (AT/AU).[39] However, a bigger study with 90 patients demonstrated a better response rate favoring patchy alopecia when compared to AT/AU (81.9% vs 59.0).[40] Also, there are results in children and adult patients.[41]

After stopping the medication, however, patient hairs started falling out again. As a consequence, treating alopecia areata (AA) patients with these small molecules should be carried out indefinitely. One option after reaching an endpoint is tapering the dose to the lowest maintenance dose. Combination therapy might be an option when tapering the dose to find the lowest dose.

Side effects

New drugs and especially, prolonged treatments always raise concern about their safety profile. These medications can potentially block important tools that act together protecting against cancer development. The most common side effects are upper respiratory and urinary tract infection. Other reported adverse events are varicella zoster, liver transaminase levels increase, serum lipid levels increase (total cholesterol, low-density lipoprotein and/or triglycerides) increase, and leukopenia/thrombocytopenia. Tuberculosis has also been reported and screened is recommended.[38,40,42]

Topical

Although mouse model studies have shown good results using topical JAK inhibitors, clinical projects treating alopecia areata patients were not as good as oral medications. The greater thickness of human skin compared with mouse models has been blamed for the poor results of topical studies. A liposomal base vehicle was tried with some benefit to deliver the necessary amount of medication. Increasing the concentration is another option that should be tried in future trials.[43–46]

SUMMARY

All the discussed treatments are promising in the area of hair loss. Patients are eager to start their protocol and see results. The long-term side effect profile, efficacy of the previously discussed treatments, initial regimen treatment, and maintenance dose, however, still need to be better evaluated.

REFERENCES

1. Kossard S. Postmenopausal frontal fibrosing alopecia. Scarring alopecia in a pattern distribution. Arch Dermatol 1994;130(6):770–4.
2. Bolduc C, Sperling LC, Shapiro J. Primary cicatricial alopecia: Lymphocytic primary cicatricial alopecias, including chronic cutaneous lupus erythematosus, lichen planopilaris, frontal fibrosing alopecia, and Graham-Little syndrome. J Am Acad Dermatol 2016;75(6):1081–99.
3. Vañó-Galván S, Molina-Ruiz AM, Serrano-Falcón C, et al. Frontal fibrosing alopecia: a multicenter review of 355 patients. J Am Acad Dermatol 2014;70(4): 670–8.
4. Moreno-Arrones OM, Saceda-Corralo D, Fonda-Pascual P, et al. Frontal fibrosing alopecia: clinical and prognostic classification. J Eur Acad Dermatol Venereol 2017;31(10):1739–45.
5. Siah TW, Shapiro J. Scarring alopecias: a trichologic emergency. Semin Cutan Med Surg 2015;34(2): 76–80.
6. Banka N, Bunagan MJK, Shapiro J. Pattern hair loss in men: diagnosis and medical treatment. Dermatol Clin 2013;31(1):129–40.
7. Fertig R, Shapiro J, Bergfeld W, et al. Investigation of the plausibility of 5-alpha-reductase inhibitor syndrome. Skin Appendage Disord 2017;2(3–4):120–9.
8. Strazzulla LC, Wang EHC, Avila L, et al. Alopecia areata - an appraisal of new treatment approaches and overview of current therapies. J Am Acad Dermatol 2018;78(1):15–24. Elsevier Inc.
9. Strazzulla LC, Wang EHC, Avila L, et al. Alopecia areata - disease characteristics, clinical evaluation, and new perspectives on pathogenesis. J Am Acad Dermatol 2018;78(1):1–12. Elsevier Inc.
10. Rakowska A, Gradzińska A, Olszewska M, et al. Efficacy of isotretinoin and acitretin in treatment of frontal fibrosing alopecia: retrospective analysis of 54 cases. J Drugs Dermatol 2017;16(10): 988–92.
11. Karnik P, Tekeste Z, McCormick TS, et al. Hair follicle stem cell-specific PPARc deletion causes scarring alopecia. J Invest Dermatol 2008;129(5):1243–57.
12. Spring P, Spanou Z, de Viragh PA. Lichen planopilaris treated by the peroxisome proliferator activated receptor-γ agonist pioglitazone: lack of lasting improvement or cure in the majority of patients. J Am Acad Dermatol 2013;69(5):830–2.
13. Baibergenova A, Walsh S. Use of pioglitazone in patients with lichen planopilaris. J Cutan Med Surg 2012;16(2):97–100.
14. Mirmirani P. Lichen planopilaris treated with a peroxisome proliferator–activated receptor γ agonist. Arch Dermatol 2009;145(12):1363.
15. Mesinkovska NA, Tellez A, Dawes D, et al. The use of oral pioglitazone in the treatment of lichen planopilaris. J Am Acad Dermatol 2015;72(2):355–6.
16. Krskova-Tybitanclova K, Macejova D, Brtko J, et al. Short term 13-cis-retinoic acid treatment at therapeutic doses elevates expression of leptin, GLUT4, PPARgamma and aP2 in rat adipose tissue. J Physiol Pharmacol 2008;59(4):731–43.
17. Alves R, Grimalt R. A review of platelet-rich plasma: history, biology, mechanism of action, and classification. Skin Appendage Disord 2018;4(1):18–24.
18. Ho A, Sukhdeo K, Sicco Lo K, et al. Trichologic response of platelet-rich plasma in androgenetic

alopecia is maintained during combination therapy. J Am Acad Dermatol 2018. [Epub ahead of print].

19. Trink A, Sorbellini E, Bezzola P, et al. A randomized, double-blind, placebo- and active-controlled, half-head study to evaluate the effects of platelet-rich plasma on alopecia areata. Br J Dermatol 2013; 169(3):690–4.

20. Bolanča Ž, Goren A, Getaldić-Švarc B, et al. Platelet-rich plasma as a novel treatment for lichen planopillaris. Dermatol Ther 2016;29(4):233–5.

21. Gupta AK, Carviel J. A mechanistic model of platelet-rich plasma treatment for androgenetic alopecia. Dermatol Surg 2016;42(12):1335–9.

22. Girijala RL, Riahi RR, Cohen PR. Platelet-rich plasma for androgenic alopecia treatment: a comprehensive review. Dermatol Online J 2018;24(7) [pii:13030/qt8s43026c].

23. Kramer ME, Keaney TC. Systematic review of platelet-rich plasma (PRP) preparation and composition for the treatment of androgenetic alopecia. J Cosmet Dermatol 2018;17(5):666–71.

24. Badran KW, Sand JP. Platelet-rich plasma for hair loss: review of methods and results. Facial Plast Surg Clin North Am 2018;26(4):469–85.

25. Amable PR, Carias RBV, Teixeira MVT, et al. Platelet-rich plasma preparation for regenerative medicine: optimization and quantification of cytokines and growth factors. Stem Cell Res Ther 2013;4(3):67.

26. Alves R, Grimalt R. Randomized placebo-controlled, double-blind, half-head study to assess the efficacy of platelet-rich plasma on the treatment of androgenetic alopecia. Dermatol Surg 2016;42(4):491–7.

27. Cervelli V, Garcovich S, Bielli A, et al. The effect of autologous activated platelet rich plasma (AA-PRP) injection on pattern hair loss: clinical and histomorphometric evaluation. Biomed Res Int 2014;2014: 760709.

28. Gentile P, Garcovich S, Bielli A, et al. The effect of platelet-rich plasma in hair regrowth: a randomized placebo-controlled trial. Stem Cells Transl Med 2015;4(11):1317–23.

29. Mapar MA, Shahriari S, Haghighizadeh MH. Efficacy of platelet-rich plasma in the treatment of androgenetic (male-patterned) alopecia: a pilot randomized controlled trial. J Cosmet Laser Ther 2016;18(8): 452–5.

30. Puig CJ, Reese R, Peters M. Double-blind, placebo-controlled pilot study on the use of platelet-rich plasma in women with female androgenetic alopecia. Dermatol Surg 2016;42(11):1243–7.

31. Ayatollahi A, Hosseini H, Shahdi M, et al. Platelet-rich plasma by single spin process in male pattern androgenetic alopecia: is it effective treatment? Indian Dermatol Online J 2017;8(6):460–4.

32. Hausauer AK, Jones DH. Evaluating the efficacy of different platelet-rich plasma regimens for management of androgenetic alopecia: a single-center, blinded, randomized clinical trial. Dermatol Surg 2018;44(9):1191–200.

33. Betz RC, Petukhova L, Ripke S, et al. Genome-wide meta-analysis in alopecia areata resolves HLA associations and reveals two new susceptibility loci. Nat Commun 2015;6:5966.

34. Petukhova L, Duvic M, Hordinsky M, et al. Genome-wide association study in alopecia areata implicates both innate and adaptive immunity. Nature 2010; 466(7302):113–7.

35. Divito SJ, Kupper TS. Inhibiting Janus kinases to treat alopecia areata. Nat Med 2014;20(9):989–90.

36. Xing L, Dai Z, Jabbari A, et al. Alopecia areata is driven by cytotoxic T lymphocytes and is reversed by JAK inhibition. Nat Med 2014;20(9):1043–9.

37. Jabbari A, Dai Z, Xing L, et al. Reversal of alopecia areata following treatment with the JAK1/2 inhibitor baricitinib. EBioMedicine 2015;2(4):351–5.

38. Wang EHC, Sallee BN, Tejeda CI, et al. JAK inhibitors for treatment of alopecia areata. J Invest Dermatol 2018;138(9):1911–6.

39. Jabbari A, Sansaricq F, Cerise J, et al. An open-label pilot study to evaluate the efficacy of tofacitinib in moderate to severe patch-type alopecia areata, totalis, and universalis. J Invest Dermatol 2018; 138(7):1539–45.

40. Liu LY, Craiglow BG, Dai F, et al. Tofacitinib for the treatment of severe alopecia areata and variants: a study of 90 patients. J Am Acad Dermatol 2017; 76(1):22–8.

41. Craiglow BG, Liu LY, King BA. Tofacitinib for the treatment of alopecia areata and variants in adolescents. J Am Acad Dermatol 2017;76(1):29–32.

42. Kennedy Crispin M, Ko JM, Craiglow BG, et al. Safety and efficacy of the JAK inhibitor tofacitinib citrate in patients with alopecia areata. JCI Insight 2016;1(15):e89776.

43. Bayart CB, DeNiro KL, Brichta L, et al. Topical Janus kinase inhibitors for the treatment of pediatric alopecia areata. J Am Acad Dermatol 2017;77(1):167–70.

44. Craiglow BG, Tavares D, King BA. Topical ruxolitinib for the treatment of alopecia universalis. JAMA Dermatol 2016;152(4):490–1.

45. Deeb M, Beach RA. A case of topical ruxolitinib treatment failure in alopecia areata. J Cutan Med Surg 2017;21(6):562–3.

46. Bokhari L, Sinclair R. Treatment of alopecia universalis with topical Janus kinase inhibitors - a double blind, placebo, and active controlled pilot study. Int J Dermatol 2018;57(12):1464–70.

What's New in Nail Disorders

Austin J. Maddy, BA*, Antonella Tosti, MD

KEYWORDS

- Nail psoriasis • Brittle nails • Onychotillomania • Retronychia • Trachyonychia

KEY POINTS

- Many changes in the diagnosis and management of nail diseases have occurred in the past years.
- It is essential that physicians be up-to-date on new diagnostic and treatment modalities to provide the best care for patients with nail complaints.
- Herein we discuss updated diagnostic and management tools for various nail disorders.

INTRODUCTION

Many changes in the diagnosis and management of nail diseases have transpired in the past years. To provide the best care for patients with nail complaints, it is essential that physicians be updated on new diagnostic and treatment modalities. The purpose of this article is to discuss new and oncoming therapeutic options for nail disorders.

NAIL PSORIASIS

Nail involvement occurs in 80% to 90% of patients with plaque psoriasis, and is even more frequent in patients with psoriatic arthritis.[1] Several biologics have been recently introduced and all have shown to be very effective. These include anti-tumor necrosis factor-α, anti–IL-17, and anti–IL-12/23.[2] Response is usually slow compared with treatment of the skin, with most noticeable improvements after approximately 12 weeks (Fig. 1).[1] Currently, it is unclear which biologic is best for nail psoriasis, because studies are difficult to compare owing to different outcome measurements.

Adalimumab is the only biologic approved by the US Food and Drug Administration with this indication. In 2017, it was approved for use in fingernail psoriasis. A recent phase III, randomized, placebo-controlled trail described at least 75% improvement on the Nail Psoriasis Severity Index (NAPSI75) in primary end point efficacy after 26 weeks of adalimumab treatment in patients with moderate to severe nail psoriasis.[3]

Apremilast, an oral small molecule inhibitor of phosphodiesterase 4, decreases the severity and extent of moderate to severe plaque psoriasis, including scalp, palmoplantar, and nail manifestations.[4] One study observed a 50% decrease in the NAPSI for 33.3% and 14.9% at 16 weeks in patients given apremilast 30 mg twice daily and placebo, respectively. At week 32, a 50% decrease in the NAPSI score response was observed in 45.2% of patients treated with apremilast in a phase III, multicenter, double-blind, placebo-controlled study.[5,6]

Tofacitinib is an oral Janus kinase inhibitor that has been shown to improve moderate to severe plaque psoriasis, as well as be an effective treatment for nail psoriasis. One study demonstrated an improvement in nail psoriasis with tofacitinib 5 and 10 mg versus placebo.[7] At week 16, significantly more patients receiving tofacitinib 5 mg and tofacitinib 10 mg versus placebo twice daily achieved NAPSI50 (32.8% and 44.2% vs 12.0%),

Disclosures: Dr A. Tosti: PI Erconia
Department of Dermatology and Cutaneous Surgery, University of Miami Miller School of Medicine, 1600 Northwest 10th Avenue #1140, Miami, FL 33136, USA
* Corresponding author. 1475 Northwest 12th Avenue, 2nd Floor, Miami, FL 33136.
E-mail address: ajm343@med.miami.edu

Dermatol Clin 37 (2019) 143–147
https://doi.org/10.1016/j.det.2018.12.004

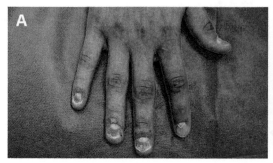
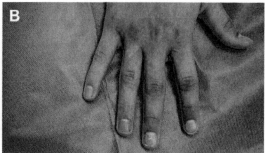

Fig. 1. (*A, B*) Nail psoriasis, Complete cure after 6 months of treatment with a tumor necrosis factor- α inhibitor.

NAPSI75 (16.9% and 28.1% vs 6.8%), and NAPSI100 (10.3% and 18.2% vs 5.1%), respectively.[7] This improvement was then maintained through week 52, suggesting that oral tofacitinib is a potentially useful agent for nail psoriasis.

CONTACT ALLERGIC AND IRRITANT REACTIONS TO ACRYLIC-BASED NAIL POLISHES

Allergic psoriasiform reactions in the nail are characterized by onycholysis and subungual hyperkeratosis of multiple fingernails (**Fig. 2**). These reactions have been reported to occur after gel nail polish manicures.[8] Psoriasiform skin lesions are also commonly associated. These patients should be patch tested with acrylates. It has been reported that 2HEMA and 2HPMA are the most commonly positive allergens.[9] Although presentation is very similar to nail psoriasis, the prognosis is very different as nail changes rapidly improve with a short course of systemic steroids associated with topical steroids (A. Tosti, unpublished data, 2018).

Pterygium inversum unguis is characterized by the abnormal adherence of the hyponychium to the ventral surface of the nail plate (**Fig. 3**). A recent case series reported 17 women who developed pterygium inversum unguis after 2 to 5 years of gel polish application.[10] Nine of 17 patients reported using both UVA and LED light to cure gel polish. Of the remaining 8, 5 used LED light only and 3 did not know or could not remember. All but 2 patients had a resolution of the disorder a few weeks after switching from gel polish to regular polish manicures.

RETRONYCHIA

Retronychia is a common but still not well-recognized traumatic nail disorder characterized by proximal nail ingrowth, with embedding of the nail plate into the proximal nail fold. It most frequently affects the great toe unilaterally, and is most common in younger patients.[11] It is associated with inflammation and swelling of the proximal nail fold, and can be very painful. The proximal nail may become opaque and thickened. Treatment for retronychia includes nail avulsion and intralesional steroids.[11,12]

BRITTLE NAILS

Although data on the efficacy of the use of biotin for brittle nails is not very strong, it is still widely

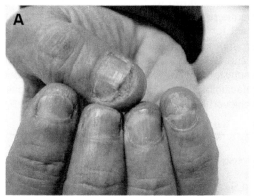
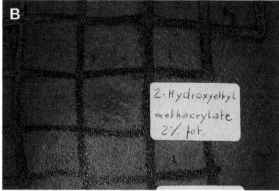

Fig. 2. (*A, B*) Psoriasiform contact dermatitis from gel polish manicure with positive patch test to 2-hydroxyethyl methacrylate.

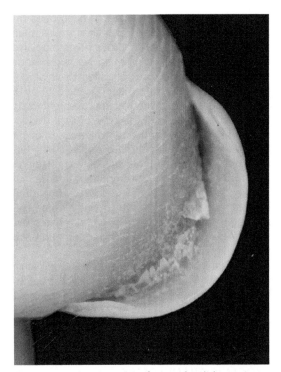

Fig. 3. Pterygium inversum from gel polish manicure.

prescribed.[13] Many dietary supplements contain biotin levels up to 650 times the recommended daily intake of 3 mg. Biotin treatments can potentially interfere with streptavidin-biotin immunoassays, because biotin in the blood may compete with biotin in the immunoassays. Exogenous biotin can also alter other markers, such as hormone tests and tests for markers of cardiac health such as troponins. Thyroid tests and prolactin tests are some of the most frequently altered studies. Pregnancy tests can also be altered.[14] Falsely low troponins may have serious implications, such as death from a myocardial infarction. It is important that patients are always informed that they should discontinue biotin treatment before having laboratory tests measured.[15] One week is typically enough, depending on dosages. Patients should also always inform health care providers of biotin and any other supplements they are taking.[14]

A recent study of 25 women with at least 1 sign of brittle nails demonstrated that daily ingestion of bioactive collagen peptides increased nail growth and improved brittle nails in conjunction with a notable decrease in the frequency of broken nails.[16]

Nail moisturizers such as petrolatum or lanolin, and humectants, such as glycerin and propylene glycol, are effective for rehydration.[17] Alpha-hydroxy acids and urea may also be used to increase the water-binding capacity of the nail plate.[18] A recent study observed hydroxypropyl-chitosan nail lacquer, when applied on the nails, is effective in improving the nail structure and appearance in subjects with brittle nails.[19] These investigators describe the efficacy of the hydroxypropyl-chitosan lacquer is specifically due to the presence of water-soluble hydroxypropyl-chitosan.

ONYCHOTILLOMANIA

Onychotillomania is common but still underdiagnosed, because it can mimic many nail disorders. Dermoscopy can be very useful, revealing features that are exclusive to this condition. We recently described wavy lines, multiple obliquely oriented nail bed hemorrhages, and nail bed gray pigmentation as diagnostic features of onychotillomania that are not seen in other nail disorders (**Fig. 4**).[20]

Wavy lines are characterized by uneven longitudinal white, reddish-purple, brown, or black pigmented lines that seem to be on different planes with a wavy appearance owing to uneven or absent nail plate growth after recurring trauma.[20] The disruption of growth leads to this bizarre and abnormal morphology that is characteristic of onychotillomania. Wavy lines can be associated with scales, hemorrhages, or nail bed pigmentation.

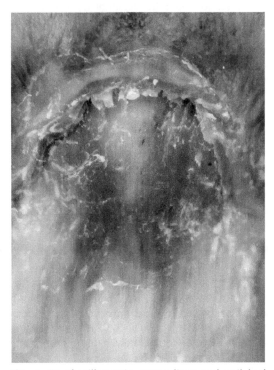

Fig. 4. Onychotillomania. Wavy lines and nail bed pigmentation.

Nail bed hemorrhages appear as reddish-brown or purplish-black streaks in the nail bed or exposed lunula area. Hemorrhages observed in onychotillomania are different from splinter hemorrhages because they are not longitudinally oriented, but instead have an oblique and wavy pattern. Nail bed pigmentation is caused by melanocyte activation owing to recurring trauma to the nail matrix and nail bed. It is associated with a loss of the nail plate. Nail bed pigmentation in onychotillomania has a gray hue on dermoscopy, which is a very distinctive feature of this disorder.[20]

Pharmacologic treatment of onychotillomania includes N-acetylcysteine at 1200 to 2400 mg/d.[21] Other remedies include manicuring or pedicuring the nails, use of occlusive dressings, and cyanoacrylate adhesives, along with behavioral modification and habit reversal training.[22,23]

TRAUMA

For permanent nail changes, such as a surgical avulsion procedure, medical tattooing (dermopigmentation) can be used to simulate reconstruction of the nail bed.[24] After anesthetizing the digital nerve with 2% lidocaine solution, a modified dermograph instrument, similar to a tattoo gun, is used to perform the procedure. One case demonstrated the use of a series of small dots rather than continuous lines of pigment to enable the treated skin area to adapt to seasonal color changes, allowing recreation of volumes and shadows to produce a 3-dimensional effect.[24] It is essential that the tattoo artist has a thorough knowledge of both nail anatomy as well as the capabilities of using the equipment.

TRACHYONYCHIA

Trachyonychia is characterized by brittle thin nails with excessive longitudinal ridging. It is most commonly associated with alopecia areata. Although these nail changes might regress spontaneously, patients with severe nail disease can seek treatment. Trachyonychia can be refractory to conventional therapies such as corticosteroids, cyclosporine, or retinoids. A recent study evaluated the efficacy and safety of oral alitretinoin for idiopathic recalcitrant trachyonychia in adults.[25] After 1, 3, and 6 months of treatment 74.3% (123/210), 98.1% (206/210), and 99.2% (119/120) of nails showed clinical improvement, respectively; 0% (0/210), 22.9% (48/210), and 69.2% (83/120) were completely free from nail abnormalities.

The efficacy of tofacitinib has also been reported.[26–28] Six patients with trachyonychia who received treatment with tofacitinib have been reported in the literature, 2 required more than 5 mg twice per day. Nail improvements may also occur even in patients who do not experience regrowth of hair. One study of patients with alopecia areata with nail involvement observed 11 of 15 patients (73.3%) who showed improvement using tofacitinib regardless of the type of nail involvement, and that nail improvements tended to occur later than hair regrowth.[29] There is no current information on the long-term benefits of the oral tofacitinib for trachyonychia. It is important to note that alopecia areata will often relapse after drug discontinuation and even during treatment. Although some studies show promising results, tofacitinib may be too aggressive of an approach for a benign disease.

A Korean study of 39 patients with idiopathic trachyonychia using calcipotriol plus betamethasone dipropionate ointment once daily to the proximal nail fold for 6 months observed complete response in 4.2% of nails and a partial response in 94.4%.[30]

PYOGENIC GRANULOMAS

Pyogenic granulomas are vascular proliferations that can affect the nail and nail folds. Treatment is typically surgical, and is usually coupled with or preceded by topical therapy.[31,32] New treatments include topical propranolol and photodynamic therapy. One study of the use of topical propranolol 1% cream observed that pyogenic granulomas owing to friction were cured, whereas pyogenic granulomas owing to chemotherapy were cured in the fingernails only. However, pyogenic granulomas owing to ingrowing toenails showed no response.[33]

Photodynamic therapy has also shown recent advancements in the treatment of pyogenic granulomas. A recent study observed complete resolution of periungual pyogenic granulomas from chemotherapy in 2 patients as well as significant improvement of clinical lesions and symptoms in 2 patients using 16% 5-methyl aminolevulinate acid for 2 hours, followed by irradiation with LED light of 635 nm. Patients went through 3 sessions every 20 days.[34]

REFERENCES

1. Pasch MC. Nail psoriasis: a review of treatment options. Drugs 2016;76(6):675–705.
2. Ortonne JP, Paul C, Berardesca E, et al. A 24-week randomized clinical trial investigating the efficacy and safety of two doses of etanercept in nail psoriasis. Br J Dermatol 2013;168(5):1080–7.

3. Elewski BE, Okun MM, Papp K, et al. Adalimumab for nail psoriasis: efficacy and safety from the first 26 weeks of a phase 3, randomized, placebo-controlled trial. J Am Acad Dermatol 2018;78(1):90–9.e1.

4. Deeks ED. Apremilast: a review in psoriasis and psoriatic arthritis. Drugs 2015;75(12):1393–403.

5. Papp K, Reich K, Leonardi CL, et al. Apremilast, an oral phosphodiesterase 4 (PDE4) inhibitor, in patients with moderate to severe plaque psoriasis: results of a phase III, randomized, controlled trial (efficacy and safety trial evaluating the effects of apremilast in psoriasis [ESTEEM] 1). J Am Acad Dermatol 2015;73(1):37–49.

6. Rich P, Gooderham M, Bachelez H, et al. Apremilast, an oral phosphodiesterase 4 inhibitor, in patients with difficult-to-treat nail and scalp psoriasis: results of 2 phase III randomized, controlled trials (ESTEEM 1 and ESTEEM 2). J Am Acad Dermatol 2016;74(1):134–42.

7. Merola JF, Elewski B, Tatulych S, et al. Efficacy of tofacitinib for the treatment of nail psoriasis: two 52-week, randomized, controlled phase 3 studies in patients with moderate-to-severe plaque psoriasis. J Am Acad Dermatol 2017;77(1):79–87.e1.

8. Mattos Simoes Mendonca M, LaSenna C, Tosti A. Severe onychodystrophy due to allergic contact dermatitis from acrylic nails. Skin Appendage Disord 2015;1(2):91–4.

9. Gonçalo M, Pinho A, Agner T, et al. Allergic contact dermatitis caused by nail acrylates in Europe. An EECDRG study. Contact Dermatitis 2018;78(4):254–60.

10. Cervantes J, Sanchez M, Eber AE, et al. Pterygium inversum unguis secondary to gel polish. J Eur Acad Dermatol Venereol 2018;32(1):160–3.

11. Poveda-Montoyo I, Vergara-de Caso E, Romero-Pérez D, et al. Retronychia a little-known cause of paronychia: a report of two cases in adolescent patients. Pediatr Dermatol 2018;35(3):e144–6.

12. Nakouri I, Litaiem N, Jones M, et al. Retronychia. J Am Podiatr Med Assoc 2018;108(1):74–6.

13. Lipner SR, Scher RK. Biotin for the treatment of nail disease: what is the evidence? J Dermatolog Treat 2018;29(4):411–4.

14. Williams GR, Cervinski MA, Nerenz RD. Assessment of biotin interference with qualitative point-of-care hCG test devices. Clin Biochem 2018;53:168–70.

15. Rigopoulos D, Elewski B, Tosti A. Is biotin safe for dermatology patients? Skin Appendage Disord 2018. https://doi.org/10.1159/000488440.

16. Hexsel D, Zague V, Schunck M, et al. Oral supplementation with specific bioactive collagen peptides improves nail growth and reduces symptoms of brittle nails. J Cosmet Dermatol 2017;16(4):520–6.

17. Iorizzo M. Tips to treat the 5 most common nail disorders. Dermatol Clin 2015;33(2):175–83.

18. Iorizzo M, Piraccini BM, Tosti A. Nail cosmetics in nail disorders. J Cosmet Dermatol 2007;6(1):53–8.

19. Sparavigna A, Caserini M, Tenconi B, et al. Effects of a novel nail lacquer based on hydroxypropyl-Chitosan (HPCH) in subjects with fingernail onychoschizia. J Dermatol Clin Res 2014;2(2):1013.

20. Maddy AJ, Tosti A. Dermoscopic features of onychotillomania: a study of 36 cases. J Am Acad Dermatol 2018. https://doi.org/10.1016/j.jaad.2018.04.015.

21. Magid M, Mennella C, Kuhn H, et al. Onychophagia and onychotillomania can be effectively managed. J Am Acad Dermatol 2017;77(5):e143–4.

22. Rieder EA, Tosti A. Onychotillomania: an underrecognized disorder. J Am Acad Dermatol 2016; 75(6):1245–50.

23. Halteh P, Scher RK, Lipner SR. Onychotillomania: diagnosis and management. Am J Clin Dermatol 2017;18(6):763–70.

24. Renzoni A, Pirrera A, Lepri A, et al. Medical tattooing, the new frontiers: a case of nail bed treatment. Ann Ist Super Sanita 2017;53(4):334–6.

25. Shin K, Kim T-W, Park S-M, et al. Alitretinoin can be a good treatment option for idiopathic recalcitrant trachyonychia in adults: an open-label study. J Eur Acad Dermatol Venereol 2018. https://doi.org/10.1111/jdv.15024.

26. Jaller JA, Jaller JJ, Jaller AM, et al. Recovery of nail dystrophy potential new therapeutic indication of tofacitinib. Clin Rheumatol 2017;36(4):971–3.

27. Ferreira SB, Scheinberg M, Steiner D, et al. Remarkable improvement of nail changes in alopecia areata universalis with 10 months of treatment with Tofacitinib: a case report. Case Rep Dermatol 2016;8(3):262–6.

28. Dhayalan A, King BA. Tofacitinib citrate for the treatment of nail dystrophy associated with alopecia universalis. JAMA Dermatol 2016;152(4):492–3.

29. Lee JS, Huh C-H, Kwon O, et al. Nail involvement in patients with moderate-to-severe alopecia areata treated with oral tofacitinib. J Dermatolog Treat 2018;1–4. https://doi.org/10.1080/09546634.2018.1466024.

30. Park J-M, Cho H-H, Kim W-J, et al. Efficacy and safety of calcipotriol/betamethasone dipropionate ointment for the treatment of trachyonychia: an open-label study. Ann Dermatol 2015;27(4):371–5.

31. Lee J, Sinno H, Tahiri Y, et al. Treatment options for cutaneous pyogenic granulomas: a review. J Plast Reconstr Aesthet Surg 2011;64(9):1216–20.

32. Piraccini BM, Bellavista S, Misciali C, et al. Periungual and subungual pyogenic granuloma. Br J Dermatol 2010;163(5):941–53.

33. Piraccini BM, Alessandrini A, Dika E, et al. Topical propranolol 1% cream for pyogenic granulomas of the nail: open-label study in 10 patients. J Eur Acad Dermatol Venereol 2016;30(5):901–2.

34. Fabbrocini G, Annunziata MC, Donnarumma M, et al. Photodynamic therapy for periungual pyogenic granuloma-like during chemotherapy: our preliminary results. Support Care Cancer 2018;26(5):1353–5.

What's New in Photoprotection
A Review of New Concepts and Controversies

Danielle G. Yeager, MD*, Henry W. Lim, MD

KEYWORDS

- Photoprotection • Photoaging • Photocarcinogenesis • Sunscreen • UV filters • Photolyases
- Antioxidants

KEY POINTS

- Recent advances, including the discovery of delayed production of cyclobutane pyrimidine dimers and biologic effects of visible light, have resulted in a more thorough understanding of the mechanisms of photodamage.
- Systemic and topical photoprotective agents, including antioxidants and photolyases, may provide additional protection against both cumulative UV radiation and visible light-induced photodamage.
- Although data are still evolving, the safety and environmental impact of organic/chemical UV filters has been questioned recently.
- Dermatologists play a pivotal role in educating patients and the public on photoprotective strategies.

INTRODUCTION

Cumulative UV radiation (UVR) exposure plays a critical role in photoaging, immunosuppression, photocarcinogenesis and the exacerbation of photodermatoses. UV-A (320–400 nm) penetrates into the dermis and damages DNA by producing reactive oxygen species.[1,2] It is the major contributor to photoaging. UV-B (290–320 nm), in contrast, is responsible for sunburns it directly damages DNA by the formation of 6-4 cyclobutane pyrimidine dimers (CPDs) and pyrimidine (6–4)pyrimidone photoproducts.[2] Both UV-A and UV-B exposure increase the risk of basal cell carcinoma, squamous cell carcinoma, and melanoma. According to the Skin Cancer Foundation, 90% of nonmelanoma skin cancers and 86% of melanomas are related to sun exposure and UVR.[2]

As a result, photoprotection is one of the most important preventative health strategies, with dermatologists playing a critical role in advising patients to implement protective measures. Photoprotection includes behavioral modifications, such as seeking shade when outdoors and wearing protective clothing, wide-brimmed hats, and sunglasses. The use of sunscreens and other products to prevent or counteract the damaging effects of UVR are also critical. Despite what is known regarding the danger of cumulative UVR exposure, adoption of these practices is not undertaken regularly by a large proportion of patients. Various obstacles exist, including

Disclosure Statement: D.G. Yeager has no conflicts of interest to disclose. H.W. Lim is an investigator/coinvestigator for Ferndale, Estee Lauder, Allergan, and Incyte. Dr Lim has served as a speaker at an education sessions organized by Pierre Fabre.
Department of Dermatology, Henry Ford Medical Center, 3031 West Grand Boulevard, Suite 800, Detroit, MI 48202, USA
* Corresponding author.
E-mail address: dyeager2@hfhs.org

Dermatol Clin 37 (2019) 149–157
https://doi.org/10.1016/j.det.2018.11.003
0733-8635/19/Published by Elsevier Inc.

lifestyle preferences and common misconceptions regarding sun protective practices. Sunscreens, which are an integral component in all photoprotective regimens, have been questioned recently in terms of their safety for users and their environmental impact. The aim of this article is to provide an overview of new concepts in photoprotection and also address current controversies pertaining to sunscreens.

NEW CONCEPTS IN PHOTOPROTECTION
Dark Cyclobutane Pyrimidine Dimers Formation

Melanin has traditionally been thought to be protective against UVR-induced DNA damage and skin cancer development. However, it has been recently found that, in a murine model, melanin may also be carcinogenic by contributing to the formation of CPDs, even after the completion of UV-A radiation. When melanin is exposed to UV-A, it induces superoxide and nitric oxide production, which causes degradation of melanin and excitation of melanin derivatives into their high-energy state.[3] It is postulated that these high-energy melanin derivatives transfer their energy to DNA, creating mutagenic CPDs hours after UV-A exposure. These CPDs that arise hours after UV exposure are referred to as delayed or "dark" CPDs. It was further shown that pheomelanin was a more potent generator of dark CPD formation than eumelanin. Although this study has not been extended to humans, it should be noted that pheomelanin is the predominant melanin in fair skinned individuals, the very skin phototype that is more prone to photocarcinogenesis.[3]

One of the benefits of the delayed formation of CPDs for up to 3 hours after UV exposure, should this occur in humans, is the opportunity for intervention during this time. A goal of future studies may be to develop products to apply after sun exposure that protect the skin. For example, in vitro, the antioxidant vitamin E has been shown to block the formation of light and dark CPDs in keratinocytes when added either before or after UV-A1 exposure.[4]

Photolyases in Sunscreens

Photolyases are enzymes that have the property of repairing CPDs. They are naturally occurring enzymes in bacteria, plants, and animals that experience high UV exposure; these enzymes are absent in humans and other placental mammals.[5] They repair DNA in the presence of flavonoids, which act as UV chromophores. After absorbing UV photons, flavonoids transfer excited electrons to the damaged DNA segments (ie, CPDs), causing

them to convert to their nucleotide monomers in preparation for their repair by photolyases.[5]

Both in vitro and in vivo studies have supported the beneficial properties of photolyases in preventing photodamage.[6–8] All human studies were done with sunscreen containing chemical (ie, organic) UV filters, with photolyases encapsulated in liposomes to enhance their penetration through stratum corneum. In another study, the efficacy of sun protection factor (SPF) 50 sunscreen, with or without antioxidants (carnosine, arazine, ergothionine) and/or photolyases in reducing CPD formation was evaluated. It was found that the combined presence of topical antioxidants and photolyases resulted in the greatest reduction in CPDs and free radical-induced protein damage compared with the sunscreen that contained either ingredient alone,[9] suggesting that antioxidants and photolyases might have a synergistic effects.[9] In patients being treated with photodynamic therapy for actinic keratoses, treatment with sunscreen containing topical photolyases resulted in longer remission times.[10,11] The use of photolyase-containing sunscreen in patients with xeroderma pigmentosum resulted in a lower incidence of new actinic keratoses, basal cell carcinomas, and squamous cell carcinomas at 1 year compared with sunscreen alone.[12] It should be noted that photolyase-containing sunscreen available in the United States at the time of writing has zinc oxide as the sole UV filter, whereas these studies were done with a product containing chemical filters.

Role of Visible Light

Historically, the focus of many photoprotection studies was on the effects of UV light. Recently, the visible light spectrum, which includes the wavelengths between 400 and 700 nm, has been found to induce skin pigmentation. UV-B–induced hyperpigmentation is attributed, in part, to increased p53 expression inducing melanogenesis. Interestingly, when compared with UV-B radiation, blue-violet light (part of the visible light spectrum) has not been found to increase p53 expression.[13] The mechanism of visible light-induced pigmentation and melanogenesis is still being actively investigated.

A study of 22 patients found that, when exposed to visible light, patients with skin types IV to VI developed darker and more sustained pigmentation compared with subjects exposed to pure UV-A1. In addition, visible light-induced pigmentation was observed up to 2 weeks after the radiation, a time point when UV-A1–induced pigmentation had resolved. These pigmentation effects were not observed in lighter skin patients of skin type II.[14] Histologic specimens in this study found that visible light-induced migration of melanin from the basal layer to the upper layers in the epidermis. This finding could explain the sustained effect of pigmentation for up to 2 weeks after visible light exposure. Visible light-induced pigmentation was irradiance dependent. Furthermore, exposure to a light source emitting visible light and a small amount of UV-A1 (0.5%) resulted in more intense pigmentation compared with exposure to pure visible light.[15]

These findings support the concept that visible light may have a role in conditions aggravated by sun exposure, such as postinflammatory hyperpigmentation and melasma, especially in darker skinned individuals. This finding is of great significance because the visible spectrum compromises 38.9% of sunlight that reaches the surface of the earth.[14] Currently available chemical (ie, organic) UV filters are not sufficient to protect the skin from the effects of visible light (**Table 1**). Similarly, current sunscreens do not provide adequate protection for the UV-A1 spectrum, which acts synergistically with visible light.[15] Although nonmicronized form of zinc oxide or titanium dioxide would physically block visible light transmission, the chalky white appearance of these agents make them aesthetically not acceptable to users. Similar to exposure to UVR, visible light exposure generates reactive oxygen species; therefore, it is possible that antioxidants could play a role in decreasing these pigmentary alterations.[16]

Vitamin D and Sunburn

UV-B is responsible for the conversion of epidermal 7-dehydrocholesterol into active vitamin D_3 (cholecalciferol), which has been found to have various immunomodulatory effects. Prior in vitro and animal studies have proven that vitamin D enhances antimicrobial responses, suppresses proinflammatory mediators, and diminishes inflammation after skin injury.[17] Recently, a pilot study of human subjects displayed that high doses of oral vitamin D_3 (cholecalciferol) are beneficial in attenuating the sunburn response. Twenty patients were randomized to receive either placebo or high doses of oral vitamin D_3 1 hour after being exposed to 3 minimal erythema doses of simulator solar radiation. compared with the placebo group, subjects who received 200,000 IU of vitamin D_3 had a sustained decrease in skin redness after the experimental sunburn with less epidermal damage noted on skin biopsies. These subjects also had a decreased release of

Table 1 Current 17 active sunscreen ingredients approved by the US Food and Drug Administration and their range of protection	
Active Ingredient/UV[a] Filter Name	**Range of Protection**
Organic (chemical) UV filters	
UV-A filters	
Avobenzone	UV-A1
Ecamsule (Mexoryl SX)[a]	UV-A2
Meradimate (menthyl anthranilate)	UV-A2
UV-B filters	
Aminobenzoic acid	UV-B
Cinoxate	UV-B
Ensulizole (phenylbenzimidazole sulfonic acid)	UV-B
Homosalate	UV-B
Octocrylene	UV-B
Octinoxate (octyl methoxycinnamate)	UV-B
Octisalate (octyl salicylate)	UV-B
Padimate	UV-B
Trolamine	UV-B
UV-A and UV-B filters	
Dioxybenzone	UV-A2, UV-B
Oxybenzone	UV-A2, UV-B
Sulisobenzone	UV-A2, UV-B
Inorganic (physical) UV filters	
Titanium dioxide	UV-A2, UV-B
Zinc oxide	UV-A1, UV-A2, UV-B

[a] Approved through New Drug Application process.

proinflammatory mediators of tumor necrosis factor-alpha and nitric oxide synthase. This finding was attributed to the upregulation of gene expression in the skin of arginase-1, which is antiinflammatory.[17] Larger clinical trials are needed to support the findings of this proof-of-concept study.

Nontopical Forms of Photoprotection

Other nontopical forms of sun protection have also been gaining interest recently to provide additional protection against UVR exposure. Sunscreens with organic and inorganic UV filters do not protect against visible light. Systemic photoprotective agents may be beneficial for these reasons.

Several studies have shown that oral and a subcutaneously administered agent have been shown to be effective in reducing photodamage, but larger studies are still needed to confirm their efficacy (**Table 2**).

Polypodium leucotomos extract is derived from a fern plant that is native in Central and South America. It has been shown to have antioxidative and antiinflammatory properties. As an antioxidant, *P leucotomos* extract decreases lipid peroxides and neutralizes superoxide anions and hydroxyl radicals after UV exposure.[18] Its antiinflammatory properties are attributed to reduced UV-induced cyclooxygenase-2 expression, p53 suppressor gene mutations, and formation of CPDs and inflammatory infiltrate in animal models.[18]

Human studies have shown that *P leucotomos* extract increases the UV dose required for immediate pigment darkening, minimal erythema dose, and minimal phototoxic dose.[19,20] It is protective against UV-B and psoralen plus UV-A–induced phototoxicity.[21] It has also been found to be beneficial in preventing polymorphous light eruption, solar urticarial, and other photodermatoses.[22] Current studies are being performed to assess its efficacy in protecting against visible light-induced delayed tanning and persistent pigment

darkening. A review of both human and basic science studies found no significant adverse effects of oral *P leucotomos* extract.[23]

Nicotinamide is the active amide form of vitamin B_3 (niacin; nicotinic acid) and is a cofactor for adenosine triphosphate, which is essential in DNA repair in the skin.[24] It is safe and widely available over the counter. Unlike niacin, it does not cause a flushing reaction. UVR typically inhibits adenosine triphosphate production and prevents optimal skin immune response and DNA repair. This pathway is ultimately responsible for photocarcinogenesis. In human keratinocytes, nicotinamide blocks the inhibitory effect of UV on adenosine triphosphate production, enhances DNA repair, and decreases the formation of CPDs.[24] In a phase II clinical trial, subjects with sun-damaged skin who took 500 mg once or twice daily had 29% and 35%, respectively, fewer actinic keratoses at 4 months.[25] A phase III trial demonstrated that nicotinamide might be beneficial as chemoprevention in subjects with a history of 2 or more nonmelanoma skin cancers. Subjects who received nicotinamide 500 mg twice daily had 23% lower rates of new nonmelanoma skin cancers and 11% fewer actinic keratosis compared with placebo at 12 months.[26] Notably, consistent with the proposed mechanism of action of

Table 2
Nontopical forms of photoprotection

Product	Source	Mechanism	Clinical Uses
Polypodium leucotomos extract	Tropical fern	Neutralization of superoxide anions, lipid peroxides and hydroxyl radicals Reduced cyclooxygenase-2 expression, p53 suppressor gene mutations, cyclobutane pyrimidine dimers, sunburn cells, and inflammatory infiltrate	Reducing immediate pigment darkening Increasing minimal erythemal dose and minimal phototoxic dose Preventing polymorphous light eruption and other photodermatoses
Nicotinamide	Active form of vitamin B_3 (niacin)	Prevent UVR-induced intracellular depletion of adenosine triphosphate Boosts cellular energy and enhances DNA repair	Chemoprevention of actinic keratosis and nonmelanoma skin cancers
Afamelanotide	Analogue of alpha-melanocyte-stimulating hormone	Stimulates eumelanin production in the epidermis without UV-induced cellular damage Results in eumelanin that absorbs UV light, reduces free radicals and reactive oxygen species	Photoprotective in patients with erythropoietic protoporphyria Possible role in polymorphous light eruption, actinic keratosis in organ transplant patients and solar urticaria

Abbreviations: UVR, UV radiation.

preventing UV-induced suppression of adenosine triphosphate production, this response is not sustained once nicotinamide is discontinued.

Afamelanotide is a structural analogue of alpha-melanocyte–stimulating hormone and acts as an agonist of melanocortin-1 receptor. It promotes the synthesis of melanin (eumelanin) without the UV-induced cellular damage that occurs with UV exposure.[27] It has been found to be photoprotective in patients with erythropoietic protoporphyria and solar urticaria by stimulating melanogenesis and acting as an antioxidant.[28,29] In phase II and phase III trials in Europe and the United States, patients with erythropoietic protoporphyria were administered 16 mg subcutaneously every 60 days; they had an improved quality of life and longer pain-free periods after sun exposure.[30] In combination with narrowband UV-B phototherapy, it has also been demonstrated to accelerate repigmentation in vitiligo.[27]

CONTROVERSIES ON SUNSCREENS
UV Blocked Versus Transmitted

SPF is a well-known term used to communicate how effective a sunscreen is in protecting against erythema-induced radiation (EIR). An incorrect misconception made by many is generalizing that SPFs beyond 30 provides only minimal additional protection.[31,32] This misconception might stem from the way that SPF is commonly presented as percent of EIR absorbed and not percent of EIR transmitted. This approach is misleading because only photons that are transmitted are absorbed and have biologic effects. For example, when comparing percent absorbed of SPF 30 with SPF 60, it is 96.7% EIR absorbed compared with 98.3% EIR absorbed. However, if comparing the number of photons transmitted when exposed to 60 photons, SPF 30 allows 2 photons to be transmitted, and SPF 60, 1 photon.

Notice that the photons transmitted are halved despite the seemingly small difference in the percent of EIR absorbed (**Table 3**).

A recent survey found that, when sunscreen SPF is presented as percent of EIR absorbed compared with percent transmitted, dermatologists underestimated the increased protection provided by the higher SPF sunscreen.[33] It is photobiologically and clinically more relevant to assess the amount of UV photons transmitted, especially in the setting of chronic sun exposure. Higher SPF sunscreens are more beneficial for long-term cumulative photoprotection.

Safety of Oxybenzone and Other Sunscreen Active Ingredients

Oxybenzone (benzophenone-3) is a widely used broad-spectrum organic filter that is protective against UV-B and UV-A2 (see **Table 1**).[34] In a 2018 report, it was estimated to be in two-thirds of nonmineral sunscreens in the United States.[34] However, concerns have been raised about its photoallergic potential, systemic absorption, endocrine side effects, and environmental impact.[35]

In 2014, benzophenones were named the American Contact Dermatitis Society's Contact Allergen of the Year. Of all the UV filters, it is the most common cause of photoallergy and contact allergy reactions.[36] In a large 10-year retrospective study, a review of the patients who listed an allergy to sunscreen found that 70.2% had a positive patch test reaction to oxybenzone.[36] In the European Union, oxybenzone has been largely replaced with other broad-spectrum UV filters. Unfortunately, this replacement cannot be easily done in the United States because many of those filters are not yet approved by the US Food and Drug Administration to be used in the United States.

Table 3
Comparison of 2 different ways to display SPF protection: percent transmitted versus percent absorbed

	% EIR Transmitted	% EIR Absorbed
SPF 1	100% transmitted × 60 photons = 60 photons transmitted	0% absorbed × 60 photons = 0 photons absorbed
SPF 15	6.7% transmitted × 60 photons = 4.02 photons transmitted	93.3% absorbed × 60 photons = 55.98 photons absorbed
SPF 30	3.3% transmitted × 60 photons = 1.98 photons transmitted	96.7% absorbed × 60 photons = 58.02 photons absorbed
SPF 60	1.7% transmitted × 60 photons = 1.02 photons transmitted	98.3% absorbed × 60 photons = 58.98 photons absorbed

Abbreviations: EIR, erythema-induced radiation; SPF, sun protection factor.
Studies have found that when SPF data are presented as %EIR absorbed, their protective effects are underestimated.

In addition, oxybenzone has been found to have endocrinologic effects in fish and rats.[37–39] In fish it has been shown to have antiandrogenic and antiestrogenic effects. Chronic exposure to oxybenzone in fish resulted in decreased egg production and egg hatchings. In rats, a dose-dependent estrogenic effect was observed when these animals were given high doses of oxybenzone ($\geq$1500 mg/kg/d) in their drinking water.[39] In humans, it has been estimated that, if one applies sunscreen at 2 mg/cm^2, which is the dose used for SPF testing, to 100% of their body surface, it would take almost 35 years of daily application to achieve the serum levels detected in rats used in that study.[40] Short-term studies that evaluated topical application of UV filters including oxybenzone in humans found that there were no significant UV filter-related alterations in endocrinologic, reproductive, or thyroid function.[40,41] It should also be emphasized

that although oxybenzone has been in used in the United States since 1978, no adverse systemic effects have been reported in humans.

There are also concerns regarding the potential for many UV filters to damaging marine environments; these filters include oxybenzone, octocrylene, octinoxate, and ethyl hexyl salicyclate.[35] In vitro, oxybenzone has shown to cause bleaching of coral reefs, inducing ossification and deforming DNA in the larval stage.[42] A study measuring the concentrations of oxybenzone in seawater in various locations, including Hawaii and the US Virgin Islands, found varying detectable levels from 0.8 µg/L to 1.4 mg/L. This study also reported that the coral cell median lethal concentration of oxybenzone for 7 different coral species ranges from 8 to 340 µg/L over 4 hours of exposure.[42] These concerns have led to Hawaii to pass a legislative bill that prohibits the sale

Table 4
Additional topical antioxidant agents

Antioxidant	Function and Use
Soy (*Glycine soja*) extract	Genistein phytoestrogen compound in soy causes dose-dependent UV-induced DNA damage and pyrimidine dimer formation.[48]
Vitamin C (L-ascorbic acid)	Topical concentrations of at least 10% are photoprotective, reducing erythema and immunosuppression. Protects from UV-B and UV-A–induced erythema and sunburn cell formation.[49]
Vitamin E (tocopherols and tocotrienols)	Protects against UV-induced lipid peroxidation, UV- induced photoaging, immunosuppression and photocarcinogenesis. Inhibits UV-induced CPD formation and inhibits melanogenesis.[49]
Grape seed extract (*Vitis vinifera*)	Inhibition of UV-mediated edema and inflammation. Inhibits inflammatory mediation cyclooxygenase-2, reduces hydrogen peroxide and causes decrease lipid peroxidation. Rapid metabolism makes it challenging for topical use unless encapsulated in lipid nanoparticles.[50]
Tea polyphenols	Epigallocatechin-3-gallate inhibits UV-B–induced release of hydrogen peroxide, and prevents phosphorylation of mitogen-activated protein kinase.[51] Reduces inflammation through nuclear factor kappa B pathway. Dose dependent inhibitor of UVR-induced erythema.[51]
Selenium	Protects against UV-induced DNA oxidation, IL-10 expression and lipid peroxidation. Protects against UV-induced erythema and skin cancer in mice. In humans, caused a dose-dependent increase in minimal erythema dose.[49]
Melatonin	Protects against UV-induced erythema, decreased production of reactive oxygen species, enhanced p53 expression, improved DNA repair and decreased CPD generation.[49]
Algae extract	Stimulates proteasome peptidase activity in irradiated human keratinocytes, reducing the extent of protein oxidative damage.[52]
Silymarin milk thistle (*Silybum marianum*)	Enhances repair of UV-B–induced DNA damage through the nucleotide excision repair pathway. Accelerates DNA repair in human dermal fibroblasts after UV-B irradiation through a p53-dependent repair pathway.[53]
Aloe vera leaf extracts	Reduces UV-A–induced redox imbalance, decrease UV-A–associated lipid membrane oxidation and increase overall cell survival.[54]

Abbreviations: CPD, cyclobutane pyrimidine dimers; UVR, UV radiation.

and distribution of oxybenzone and octinoxate. The bill was signed into law by the governor on July 3, 2018, and will take effect in January 2021.

Nanoparticle Free Radical Damage to the Skin

The safety of broad-spectrum inorganic UV filters or physical sunscreens, titanium dioxide, and zinc oxide has also been questioned. Titanium oxide and zinc oxide are formulated as nanosized products that blend more easily into the skin. When exposed to UV light in vitro, titanium oxide and zinc oxide emit electrons and generate free radicals and reactive oxygen species.[43] The major concern is that, when exposed to UVR, these nanoparticles may have the potential to damage proteins, lipids, and DNA. It should be noted that all nanoparticles used in sunscreens are coated (usually with silica), greatly limiting the amount of free radicals that are released into the microenvironment. Furthermore, many studies have found that these nanoparticles do not penetrate through intact healthy skin and are mostly limited to the stratum corneum.[44] One recent study using porcine skin found that UV-B–damaged skin slightly enhanced both titanium and zinc oxide penetration into the epidermis but no transdermal or systemic absorption was seen.[44] Additionally, toxicity studies of titanium oxide and zinc oxide nanoparticles used subcutaneous and intravenous administration and showed low general toxicity.[45]

Antioxidants in Sunscreen

Sunscreens containing topical antioxidants have been found to reduce the production of reactive oxygen species, cytokines, and matrix metalloproteinase-1 expression after irradiation by UV and visible light.[16] Combining broad-spectrum sunscreen with antioxidants has been found to be superior to just sunscreen alone in suppressing UV-induced pigmentation, depletion of Langerhan cells, and induction of matrix metalloproteinases.[46,47] However, topical antioxidants are limited by their diffusion into the epidermis and their stability. Incorporation of stabilized antioxidants into sunscreens has gained popularity recently among pharmaceutical and cosmeceutical companies (**Table 4**).[48–54]

SUMMARY

Recent advances in photomedicine, including the discovery of delayed production of CPDs and biologic effects of visible light, have resulted in a more thorough understanding of the mechanisms of photodamage. These discoveries open the door for additional therapeutic options, including systemic photoprotective agents and additional topical agents including antioxidants and photolyases. Proper education of the public should continue to be done on photoprotection, which includes seeking shade when outdoors, wearing photoprotective clothing, wide brimmed hats and sunglasses and applying broad spectrum, with an SPF 30 or greater sunscreen. Although data are still evolving, for those who are concerned about the environmental impact of organic/chemical UV filters, sunscreens with inorganic/physical filters can be used.

REFERENCES

1. Wang SQ, Balagula Y, Osterwalder U. Photoprotection: a review of the current and future technologies. Dermatol Ther 2010;23:31–47.
2. Cohen LE, Grant RT. Sun protection: current management strategies addressing UV exposure. Clin Plast Surg 2016;43:605–10.
3. Premi S, Wallisch S, Mano CM, et al. Photochemistry. Chemiexcitation of melanin derivatives induces DNA photoproducts long after UV exposure. Science 2015;347:842–7.
4. Delinasios GJ, Karbaschi M, Cooke MS, et al. Vitamin E inhibits the UVAI induction of "light" and "dark" cyclobutane pyrimidine dimers, and oxidatively generated DNA damage, in keratinocytes. Sci Rep 2018;8:423.
5. Bhatia N, Berman B, Ceilley RI, et al. Understanding the role of photolyases: photoprotection and beyond. J Drugs Dermatol 2017;16:61–6.
6. Kabir Y, Seidel R, McKnight B, et al. DNA repair enzymes: an important role in skin cancer prevention and reversal of photodamage–a review of the literature. J Drugs Dermatol 2015;14:297–303.
7. Grewe M, Stege H, Vink A, et al. Inhibition of intercellular adhesion molecule-1 (ICAM-1) expression in ultraviolet B-irradiated human antigen-presenting cells is restored after repair of cyclobutane pyrimidine dimers. Exp Dermatol 2000;9:423–30.
8. Stege H, Roza L, Vink AA, et al. Enzyme plus light therapy to repair DNA damage in ultraviolet-B-irradiated human skin. Proc Natl Acad Sci U S A 2000;97:1790–5.
9. Emanuele E, Spencer JM, Braun M. An experimental double-blind irradiation study of a novel topical product (TPF 50) compared to other topical products with DNA repair enzymes, antioxidants, and growth factors with sunscreens: implications for preventing skin aging and cancer. J Drugs Dermatol 2014;13:309–14.
10. Puig S, Puig-Butille JA, Diaz MA, et al. Field cancerisation improvement with topical application of a film-forming medical device containing photolyase

and UV filters in patients with actinic keratosis, a pilot study. J Clin Exp Dermatol Res 2014;5:220.

11. Eibenschutz L, Silipo V, De Simone P, et al. A 9-month, randomized, assessor-blinded, parallel-group study to evaluate clinical effects of film-forming medical devices containing photolyase and sun filters in the treatment of field cancerization compared with sunscreen in patients after successful photodynamic therapy for actinic keratosis. Br J Dermatol 2016;175:1391–3.

12. Giustini S, Miraglia E, Berardesca E, et al. Preventive long-term effects of a topical film-forming medical device with ultra-high UV protection filters and DNA repair enzyme in xeroderma pigmentosum: a retrospective study of eight cases. Case Rep Dermatol 2014;6:222–6.

13. Duteil L, Cardot-Leccia N, Queille-Roussel C, et al. Differences in visible light-induced pigmentation according to wavelengths: a clinical and histological study in comparison with UVB exposure. Pigment Cell Melanoma Res 2014;27:822–6.

14. Mahmoud BH, Ruvolo E, Hexsel CL, et al. Impact of long-wavelength UVA and visible light on melano-competent skin. J Invest Dermatol 2010;130:2092–7.

15. Kohli I, Chaowattanapanit S, Mohammad TF, et al. Synergistic effects of long-wavelength ultraviolet A1 and visible light on pigmentation and erythema. Br J Dermatol 2018;178:1173–80.

16. Liebel F, Kaur S, Ruvolo E, et al. Irradiation of skin with visible light induces reactive oxygen species and matrix-degrading enzymes. J Invest Dermatol 2012;132:1901–7.

17. Scott JF, Das LM, Ahsanuddin S, et al. Oral vitamin D rapidly attenuates inflammation from sunburn: an interventional study. J Invest Dermatol 2017;137:2078–86.

18. Middelkamp-Hup MA, Pathak MA, Parrado C, et al. Oral Polypodium leucotomos extract decreases ultraviolet-induced damage of human skin. J Am Acad Dermatol 2004;51:910–8.

19. Choudhry SZ, Bhatia N, Ceilley R, et al. Role of oral Polypodium leucotomos extract in dermatologic diseases: a review of the literature. J Drugs Dermatol 2014;13:148–53.

20. Nestor MS, Berman B, Swenson N. Safety and efficacy of oral polypodium leucotomos extract in healthy adult subjects. J Clin Aesthet Dermatol 2015;8:19–23.

21. Middelkamp-Hup MA, Pathak MA, Parrado C, et al. Orally administered Polypodium leucotomos extract decreases psoralen-UVA-induced phototoxicity, pigmentation, and damage of human skin. J Am Acad Dermatol 2004;50:41–9.

22. Caccialanza M, Recalcati S, Piccinno R. Oral polypodium leucotomos extract photoprotective activity in 57 patients with idiopathic photodermatoses. G Ital Dermatol Venereol 2011;146:85–7.

23. Winkelmann RR, Del Rosso J, Rigel DS. Polypodium leucotomos extract: a status report on clinical efficacy and safety. J Drugs Dermatol 2015;14:254–61.

24. Lim HW, Arellano-Mendoza MI, Stengel F. Current challenges in photoprotection. J Am Acad Dermatol 2017;76:S91–9.

25. Surjana D, Halliday GM, Martin AJ, et al. Oral nicotinamide reduces actinic keratoses in phase II double-blinded randomized controlled trials. J Invest Dermatol 2012;132:1497–500.

26. Chen AC, Martin AJ, Choy B, et al. A phase 3 randomized trial of nicotinamide for skin-cancer chemoprevention. N Engl J Med 2015;373:1618–26.

27. Lim HW, Grimes PE, Agbai O, et al. Afamelanotide and narrowband UVB for the treatment of vitiligo: a randomized, multicenter trial. JAMA Dermatol 2015;151(1):42–50.

28. Harms J, Lautenschlager S, Minder CE, et al. An alpha-melanocyte-stimulating hormone analogue in erythropoietic protoporphyria. N Engl J Med 2009; 360:306–7.

29. Haylett AK, Nie Z, Brownrigg M, et al. Systemic photoprotection in solar urticaria with alpha-melanocyte-stimulating hormone analogue [Nle4-D-Phe7]-alpha-MSH. Br J Dermatol 2011;164:407–14.

30. Langendonk JG, Balwani M, Anderson KE, et al. Afamelanotide for erythropoietic protoporphyria. N Engl J Med 2015;373:48–59.

31. Your burning questions, answered. Our scientific sunscreen testing exposes startling truths about product claims and effectiveness. Consum Rep 2016;81:21–9.

32. Craven McGinty J. What SPF really means: sunscreens' perplexing figures. In: Wall St J. Available at: http://online.wsj.com/public/resources/documents/print/WSJ_-A002-20150711.pdf. Accessed July 6, 2018.

33. Herzog SM, Lim HW, Williams MS, et al. Sun protection factor communication of sunscreen effectiveness: a web-based study of perception of effectiveness by dermatologists. JAMA Dermatol 2017;153:348–50.

34. The trouble with ingredients in sunscreens. Environmental Working Group's guide to sunscreens website. Available at: https://www.ewg.org/sunscreen/report/the-trouble-with-sunscreen-chemicals/#.W24jrC2ZOog. Accessed August 13, 2018.

35. Schneider SL, Lim HW. Review of environmental effects of oxybenzone and other sunscreen active ingredients. J Am Acad Dermatol 2018. https://doi.org/10.1016/j.jaad.2018.06.033.

36. Warshaw EM, Wang MZ, Maibach HI, et al. Patch test reactions associated with sunscreen products and the importance of testing to an expanded series: retrospective analysis of North American Contact Dermatitis Group data, 2001 to 2010. Dermatitis 2013;24:176–82.

37. Ma R, Cotton B, Lichtensteiger W, et al. UV filters with antagonistic action at androgen receptors in the MDA-kb2 cell transcriptional-activation assay. Toxicol Sci 2003;74:43–50.

38. Heneweer M, Muusse M, van den Berg M, et al. Additive estrogenic effects of mixtures of frequently used UV filters on pS2-gene transcription in MCF-7 cells. Toxicol Appl Pharmacol 2005;208:170–7.

39. Schlumpf M, Cotton B, Conscience M, et al. In vitro and in vivo estrogenicity of UV screens. Environ Health Perspect 2001;109:239–44.

40. Wang SQ, Burnett ME, Lim HW. Safety of oxybenzone: putting numbers into perspective. Arch Dermatol 2011;147:865–6.

41. Janjua NR, Mogensen B, Andersson AM, et al. Systemic absorption of the sunscreens benzophenone-3, octyl-methoxycinnamate, and 3-(4-methyl-benzylidene) camphor after whole-body topical application and reproductive hormone levels in humans. J Invest Dermatol 2004;123:57–61.

42. Downs CA, Kramarsky-Winter E, Segal R, et al. Toxicopathological effects of the sunscreen UV filter, oxybenzone (benzophenone-3), on coral planulae and cultured primary cells and its environmental contamination in Hawaii and the U.S. Virgin Islands. Arch Environ Contam Toxicol 2016;70:265–88.

43. Newman MD, Stotland M, Ellis JI. The safety of nano-sized particles in titanium dioxide- and zinc oxide-based sunscreens. J Am Acad Dermatol 2009;61: 685–92.

44. Monteiro-Riviere NA, Wiench K, Landsiedel R, et al. Safety evaluation of sunscreen formulations containing titanium dioxide and zinc oxide nanoparticles in UVB sunburned skin: an in vitro and in vivo study. Toxicol Sci 2011;123:264–80.

45. Fabian E, Landsiedel R, Ma-Hock L, et al. Tissue distribution and toxicity of intravenously administered titanium dioxide nanoparticles in rats. Arch Toxicol 2008;82:151–7.

46. Wu Y, Matsui MS, Chen JZ, et al. Antioxidants add protection to a broad-spectrum sunscreen. Clin Exp Dermatol 2011;36:178–87.

47. Grether- Beck S, Marini A, Jaenicke T, et al. Effective photoprotection of human skin against infrared A radiation by topically applied antioxidants: results from a vehicle controlled, double-blind, randomized study. Photochem Photobiol 2015;91:248–50.

48. Pinnell SR. Cutaneous photodamage, oxidative stress, and topical antioxidant protection. J Am Acad Dermatol 2003;48:1–19 [quiz: 20–2].

49. Dunaway S, Odin R, Zhou L, et al. Natural antioxidants: multiple mechanisms to protect skin from solar radiation. Front Pharmacol 2018;9:392.

50. Heinrich U, Moore CE, De Spirt S, et al. Green tea polyphenols provide photoprotection, increase microcirculation, and modulate skin properties of women. J Nutr 2011;141:1202–8.

51. Afaq F, Adhami VM, Ahmad N, et al. Inhibition of ultraviolet B-mediated activation of nuclear factor kappaB in normal human epidermal keratinocytes by green tea Constituent (-)-epigallocatechin-3-gallate. Oncogene 2003;22:1035–44.

52. Hyun YJ, Piao MJ, Ko MH, et al. Photoprotective effect of Undaria crenata against ultraviolet B-induced damage to keratinocytes. J Biosci Bioeng 2013;116: 256–64.

53. Guillermo-Lagae R, Deep G, Ting H, et al. Silibinin enhances the repair of ultraviolet B-induced DNA damage by activating p53-dependent nucleotide excision repair mechanism in human dermal fibroblasts. Oncotarget 2015;6:39594–606.

54. Rodrigues D, Viotto AC, Checchia R, et al. Mechanism of Aloe Vera extract protection against UVA: shelter of lysosomal membrane avoids photodamage. Photochem Photobiol Sci 2016;15:334–50.

What's New in Melanoma

Giselle Prado, MD[a],*, Ryan M. Svoboda, MD, MS[b,1], Darrell S. Rigel, MD, MS[c]

KEYWORDS

- Melanoma epidemiology • Risk factors • Diagnosis • Prognosis • Management • Genomics

KEY POINTS

- The incidence of melanoma continues to increase, with a lifetime risk of 1 in 24 persons developing melanoma, but mortalities are decreasing because of increased awareness, early detection, and the availability of targeted therapies for advanced tumors.
- Primary prevention efforts to decrease the incidence of melanoma through behavior changes are less effective than secondary prevention efforts directed at early detection.
- Researchers continue to elucidate the myriad risk factors that predispose individuals to melanoma, including inflammatory bowel disease, phosphodiesterase-5 use, and pregnancy-diagnosed melanoma.
- Genomics and noninvasive devices are revolutionizing clinical management of melanoma, specifically through gene expression.
- Combination targeted therapies (double and triple pathway inhibition) are now being used to treat advanced melanoma.

INTRODUCTION

Issues related to melanoma are some of the most dynamic within dermatology (**Fig. 1**). Recent discoveries and new technologies have led to major advances in the diagnosis, management, and treatment of this cancer. As the incidence of melanoma continues to increase, understanding and applying these new approaches in the clinical setting has become increasingly important. From deciding whether to biopsy a suspicious pigmented lesion, to making an accurate diagnosis of an uncertain histopathologic presentation, to using genomics to better assess diagnosis and prognosis, to selectively targeting immune checkpoints that are dysregulated in melanoma, the management of melanoma has advanced greatly in the past few years. A comprehensive understanding of these issues is critical for dermatologists in the clinical setting.

EPIDEMIOLOGY

In the United States, there will be more than 90,000 cases of invasive melanoma and more than 87,000 cases of melanoma in situ diagnosed in 2018.[1] This incidence yields a lifetime risk of 1 in 24 persons for developing any type of melanoma. Among reported cancers, melanoma is the fifth most common in men and sixth most common in women.[2] Men are at a 40% increased risk to develop invasive melanoma in their lifetimes compared with women.[1]

Melanoma is one of the few cancers in the United States for which the incidence continues to increase. The lifetime risk of invasive melanoma in the United States has tripled from 1985 to 2018 and is projected to continue increasing.[1] Similarly, melanoma incidence has been increasing worldwide.[3]

Melanoma remains the deadliest form of skin cancer, accounting for 70% of skin cancer deaths.

Disclosure: Dr D.S. Rigel serves on advisory boards with Castle, DermTech, and Myriad.
[a] National Society for Cutaneous Medicine, 35 East 35th Street #208, New York, NY 10016, USA; [b] Department of Dermatology, Duke University School of Medicine, Durham, NC, USA; [c] Department of Dermatology, NYU School of Medicine, 35 East 35th Street #208, New York, NY 10016, USA
[1] Present address: 400 Ivy Meadow Lane, Apartment 2A, Durham, NC 27707.
* Corresponding author.
E-mail address: drgiselleprado@gmail.com

Dermatol Clin 37 (2019) 159–168
https://doi.org/10.1016/j.det.2018.12.005
0733-8635/19/© 2018 Elsevier Inc. All rights reserved.

derm.theclinics.com

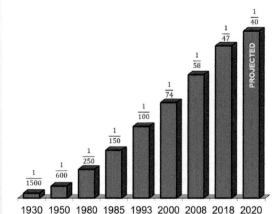

Fig. 1. Lifetime risk of invasive melanoma in the United States from 1930 to a projected risk in 2020.

More than 1 American dies from melanoma every hour. However, because of earlier detection and more effective treatments for melanoma, the absolute number of deaths in the United States has been decreasing since 2017 after peaking at about 10,000 in 2016.[4]

RISK FACTORS

Ultraviolet (UV) exposure and genetic predisposition (skin phenotype) remain the most important risk factors for the development of melanoma.[5–7] However, recent studies have shown other factors that may be contributory to melanoma risk.

Studies researching the effect of aspirin or nonsteroidal antiinflammatory drugs (NSAIDs) on melanoma have had conflicting results.[8] Five studies showed a protective effect of aspirin and NSAID use on melanoma, whereas 4 studies showed no protective effect. Given the proven beneficial effects on cardiovascular health and colon cancer, daily aspirin or NSAID use may be beneficial for patients with an increased risk of melanoma, such as patients with dysplastic nevus syndrome or positive family history. A more recent study of 1522 patients with melanoma found that aspirin use was associated with longer overall survival in patients with stage 2 and 3 melanoma.[9] This finding warrants future clinical trials to investigate the therapeutic potential of aspirin in patients with melanoma.

Coffee has also been purported to be chemopreventive in melanoma. A meta-analysis of 7 studies found that higher coffee consumption was associated with a 0.8 times reduced risk of melanoma.[10] Decaffeinated coffee was not found to have the same effect. Another meta-analysis of 23 studies encompassing more than 2 million participants found the same effect: the persons

with the highest levels of coffee consumption had a lower melanoma risk.[11] The investigators reported a dose-response relationship between coffee consumption and melanoma risk in which an increase in 1 cup of coffee per day resulted in a 3% decrease in melanoma risk.

Inflammatory bowel disease (IBD) has been associated with an increased risk of melanoma. In a recent meta-analysis of 12 studies comprising 172,837 patients with IBD, the investigators found a 37% increased risk of melanoma.[12] This rate was consistent among both Crohn disease and ulcerative colitis.

Phosphodiesterase-5 inhibitor use has been associated with an increased risk of developing melanoma. A meta-analysis of 5 observational studies found a slightly increased risk (odds ratio, 1.12).[13] However, there were no prospective studies available for analysis to confirm the association.

Women who are diagnosed with melanoma during pregnancy are at increased risk for recurrence. In a study of 462 women less than 49 years old with a history of melanoma, pregnancy-associated melanoma was associated with a 9 times increased risk of recurrence, a 7 times increased risk of metastasis, and a 5 times risk of mortality.[14] It is recommended that patients diagnosed with melanoma during pregnancy or within 1 year of childbirth be followed more closely.

The association between vitamin D level and melanoma has also been studied. A study of 1191 patients followed for 11 years found that a higher baseline vitamin D level was associated with a 2.7 times increased risk for melanoma.[15] The investigators concluded that the carcinogenicity of high sun exposure cannot be counteracted by higher vitamin D levels. Therefore, increasing vitamin D levels should be accomplished by dietary supplementation instead of through sun exposure.

PREVENTION

Primary prevention of skin cancer (behavioral changes) affects the incidence of melanoma, whereas secondary prevention (early detection efforts) affects the mortality. Based on the epidemiologic data presented earlier, secondary prevention seems to be making an impact through decreased mortality of melanoma, whereas primary prevention efforts have not led to a decreased number of cases at this point.

Behavioral change can lead to reduced risk for the development of this cancer. A primary prevention campaign directed at student athletes found that, after an educational intervention, the participants were more likely to use sunscreen 4 or more times per week, recognize their increased risk of skin cancer, and participate in discussions about sun safety with coaches.[16]

Earlier detection initiatives can also lead to improved mortality. A secondary prevention effort that increased the early detection of melanoma among women undergoing mammography seemed to achieve its desired outcome.[17] Educational materials about skin self-examination were placed in changing rooms of mammography clinics. Most women noticed the materials on their own and were able to identify at least 1 personal risk factor for melanoma. After seeing the materials, 20% of the women performed a skin self-examination in the changing room and, of these, 13% noticed a concerning mole and most intended to follow up with a dermatologist.

As discussed earlier, patients with melanoma are more likely to develop further melanomas. Targeting these patients for preventive interventions is of high importance. A systematic review of behavioral intervention techniques for high-risk patients with melanoma found that most interventions resulted in increased photoprotective behaviors among participants, such as wearing protective clothing and engaging in skin self-examination.[18]

For these high-risk patients, the skin self-examination can mean the difference between life and death. However, it is difficult to examine the entire body surface area without a partner. Organizations such as the American Academy of Dermatology have advanced Check Your Partner campaigns to address this obstacle to skin self-examination.[19] A clinical trial of 494 patient-partner couples randomized to skin self-examination training or control showed that the training increased the frequency of examinations reported throughout the 2-year study period.[20]

Sunscreen

Regular sunscreen use decreases melanoma risk.[21,22] There has been long-standing debate over whether higher sun protection factor (SPF) sunscreens protect against UV radiation more than sunscreens with lower SPF. Opponents claims that increased SPF can lead to a false sense of security among users and increased time spent in the sun. Supporters argue that increased SPF makes up for the low concentrations of sunscreen applied by the average sunscreen user.

Controversy exists regarding the questions of whether there should there be a cap of 50+ on sunscreen SPFs (**Table 1**). Proponents suggest that higher SPFs cost disproportionately more, higher values seem to have disproportionally higher protection, and higher SPF sunscreens have higher concentrations of sunscreening agents that may lead to increased allergic reactions. Opponents cite the facts that people under-apply sunscreens so higher SPFs are more forgiving at real-world application levels, that fair-skinned persons or those in high-insolation environments are not able to determine whether 50+ sunscreens are 51 or significantly higher, and that there will be no incentive to research and develop more protective sunscreens if manufacturers will not get credit. Almost half of the world currently has a 50+ cap, whereas the remaining countries do not.

In an attempt to help settle this issue, a double-blind randomized controlled trial of 199 patients showed that SPF 100+ is more effective at protecting against sunburn than SPF 50+ in real-world conditions in all skin types.[23] The results of the split-face study showed that the side randomized to SPF 50+ was 11 times more likely to be sunburned than the SPF 100+ side. The participants used the same amounts of sunscreen and reapplied equally on both sides. Even when analyzing for number of reapplications and

Table 1	
Benefits and disadvantages of capping sunscreen sun protection factors at 50+	
Benefits	Disadvantages
• Above SPF 50, doubling SPF values only results in a very small marginal additional protection	• Higher SPF sunscreens still can provide reasonable protection when underapplied at typically used concentrations
• Lower cost of sunscreens because higher SPF sunscreen is disproportionately more expensive	• No ability to discern between SPF 51 and higher SPFs for persons who may need greater protection
• Potentially fewer allergic reactions caused by lower concentrations of sunscreening agents	• No incentive for manufacturers to develop higher SPF sunscreens because no credit will be recognized
• More uniform reporting of SPF by manufacturers	• Decreased sun protection will be available to patients, potentially leading to increased skin cancer
• Less variability in claims about sunscreens	

Fitzpatrick skin type, higher SPF was still more protective.

Extensive controversy has recently unfolded over the inclusion of oxybenzone in sunscreen. Hawaii went as far as to ban the ingredient in sunscreens purchased in that state because of concerns about environmental toxicity to coral. Oxybenzone has been mired in controversy for a long time because of nonhuman studies that found estrogenic effects in the uteruses of rats. However, none of the evidence cited against oxybenzone has been found in humans or in conditions reflective of marine environments.[24] At present, the risk is entirely theoretic, but a ban on a key sunscreen ingredient will be sure to have long-lasting effects on skin cancer rates.

Complementary Sun Protection Supplements

Catechins, ingredients found in green tea, have been purported to decrease direct DNA damage induced by solar radiation. However, a double-blind randomized controlled trial in 50 patients receiving an oral green tea catechin extract with vitamin C or placebo did not find a significant difference in the number of cyclobutane pyrimidine dimer–positive cells in epidermis irradiated with UV.[25]

Polypodium leucotomos (PL) is a fern native to South America that is used for its antioxidant and photoprotective properties. The extract from this plant does not act as a sunscreen but has been shown to have some photoprotective efficacy. A recent systematic review of the clinical safety and efficacy of PL extract included 18 human studies to support its use as an additional sun-protective measure.[26] There were no reported serious adverse effects and the most commonly reported side effect was mild gastrointestinal discomfort.

Future prevention efforts should focus on preventing new melanomas through both primary and secondary prevention initiatives. To be effective there must be a comprehensive approach including UV protection (sunscreen, UV-blocking clothing, avoiding the midday sun), thereby minimizing the number of lifetime sunburns and initiatives that facilitate earlier detection through increased awareness and better access to dermatologic care.

DIAGNOSIS
Diagnostic Devices

Electrical impedance spectroscopy
The accuracy of clinical diagnosis in melanoma using the unaided human eye alone is about 70%.[27] Novel diagnostic devices are paving the way for the noninvasive diagnosis of melanoma. One such device uses electrical impedance spectroscopy (EIS) to generate an EIS score that reflects the degree of cellular atypia in pigmented lesions (Nevisense, SciBase AB, Stockholm, Sweden). The device uses a handheld probe with a disposable electrode to measure the electrical impedance of a lesion. The pins on the end of the probe penetrate to the level of the stratum corneum to perform the procedure. This screening device is highly sensitive (97%) and has a specificity of 34% compared with histopathology.[28]

Ultrasonography
High-frequency ultrasonography can be used to evaluate the epidermal, subdermal, and subcutaneous tissues in real time.[29] However, this technology is both operator and equipment dependent for interpretation of results. It can be used to diagnose melanocytic skin lesions and subclinical metastatic foci near the lesion, which can facilitate the physician's decision to pursue further histopathologic analysis. Using the knowledge of lesion borders, volume, and depth can help clinicians minimize tissue loss and improve cosmetic outcomes.

Confocal microscopy
In vivo confocal microscopy can be a helpful adjunct to visual examination in diagnosing melanoma. In a study of 857 lesions, the addition of confocal scanning laser microscopy resulted in 96% and 97% correctly classified benign and malignant lesions, respectively,[30] compared with 80% benign and 85% malignant correctly classified lesions with visual examination alone.

GENOMICS IN MELANOMA DIAGNOSIS AND PROGNOSIS
Genomics in Decision to Biopsy

Clinically suspicious pigmented lesions have traditionally been sent for definitive diagnosis with biopsy. However, for patients with many suspicious nevi or nevi in cosmetically sensitive areas, biopsy is not always easily possible or accepted by patients.

A noninvasive genetic test has been developed that samples skin cells harvested by an adhesive patch for expression of 2 genes (Pigmented Lesion Assay, DermTech, La Jolla, CA)[31,32] (**Table 2**). The genetic material undergoes quantitative reverse transcriptase polymerase chain reaction (RT-PCR) and RNA expression levels of long intergenic non–protein-coding RNA 518 (LINC00518) and melanoma antigen preferentially expressed in tumors (PRAME) are determined. The test yields a low-risk, moderate-risk, or high-risk result for

Table 2
Genomic testing for melanoma

Clinical Query	Available Test
Diagnosis: decision to biopsy	2 GEP
Diagnosis: ambiguous lesions under light microscopy	23 GEP
Prognosis: risk of metastasis in 5 y ears	31 GEP

Abbreviation: GEP, gene expression profile.

each lesion. In line with other screening tests, this test has a high sensitivity of 91% and a specificity of 69% for melanoma.[31]

Genomics in Histopathologically Ambiguous Lesions

Melanomas can show a wide variety of histopathologic characteristics that may overlap with benign melanocytic lesions. In difficult cases, dermatopathologists now have the ability to order a 23 gene expression profile (GEP) test to differentiate benign from malignant melanocytic lesions (myPath Melanoma, Myriad Genetics, Salt Lake City, UT) (see **Table 2**).[33–35] The test analyzes the RNA expression of 23 genes within sample tissue. The test can be done with existing biopsy material and determines an outcome of benign, indeterminate, or malignant. The test has a sensitivity of 90% to 94% and a specificity of 91% to 96%. Studies have shown that this test increases definitive diagnoses and affects patient management decisions.[36,37]

Stage at Diagnosis

An analysis of 26,958 patients with melanoma in the Ohio Cancer Incidence Surveillance system found that black patients are 3 times more likely to present with stage 3 or 4 disease.[38] This rate may be caused by a lower index of suspicion for melanoma by these patients and physicians leading to a delay in diagnosis. Similarly, type of insurance significantly influenced the stage at diagnosis, with Medicaid patients twice as likely to present at higher stage than private insurance patients. This trend held for patients with Medicare and uninsured patients.

Reporting of Melanoma to Cancer Registries

All US states mandate reporting of melanoma to centralized cancer registries. However, physicians may not be aware of the reporting requirements or may choose not to comply with these mandates. A survey of 158 dermatologists found that only 34% of respondents routinely report newly diagnosed

melanoma cases.[39] Less experienced practitioners and those who rarely encountered patients with melanoma in their practices were both less aware of reporting mandates and less likely to report cases if they were aware.

Surprisingly, when comparing the results of the 2017 study to a similar study conducted in 2010, respondents had lower rates of reporting to registries (44% in 2010 and 34% in 2017).[40] This widespread underreporting of melanoma may lead to significant underestimates of true incidence with resulting implications for resource allocation.

PROGNOSIS
Sentinel Lymph Node Status

Although tumor thickness is the most significant prognostic factor in melanoma, sentinel lymph node biopsy (SLNBx) status has been shown to be more significant in some models. However, the impact on survival of patients undergoing the procedure as well as its ability to alone fully predict survival remains controversial.

SLNBx has been associated with improved survival in some studies[41,42] and has been extensively criticized by other investigators.[43] A clinical trial of 1934 SLNBx-positive patients with melanoma randomized participants to completion lymph node dissection or nodal observation with ultrasonography.[44] The mean melanoma-specific survival rates at 3 years were similar in both groups. Although disease-free survival was slightly higher in the dissection group (68 months vs 63 months), patients in the dissection group developed lymphedema more often than those in the observation group. Therefore, completion dissection can control the regional disease but may not increase survival.

Genomics for Prognosis

A 31-GEP test has been developed for classifying patients with invasive melanoma into low risk and high risk for metastasis at 5 years (DecisionDx Melanoma, Castle Biosciences, Friendswood, TX) (see **Table 2**). This test uses RT-PCR to determine the differential expression of 31 genes (28 prognostic and 3 control genes) that vary in nonmetastatic and metastatic melanoma lesions. The test results (from low to high risk) are as follows: class 1a, class 1b, class 2a, and class 2b. The test does not require special processing of sample tissue and can be run on the primary biopsy specimen.

This test has been validated by multiple retrospective and prospective studies. The studies have consistently shown high sensitivity for recurrence, distant metastasis-free survival, and overall survival.[45–47] One study of 256 patients who underwent 31-GEP testing found a negative predictive value of 99%, sensitivity of 77%, and specificity of 87%.[46] The 31-GEP test has also been shown to affect clinical management in the direction dictated by the test results (eg, higher-risk patients undergo more frequent follow-up, imaging, and laboratory testing).[48–50]

Adding the information obtained from the 31-GEP test to SLNBx status seems to significantly improve prognostic assessment.[51] Given that there are so many more SLNBx-negative patients, the absolute number of patients who die from melanomas that are SLNBx negative is greater than for those that are SLNBx positive. When used in SLNBx-negative patients, the 31-GEP test has been shown to identify most of those who subsequently develop distant metastatic disease.[51] Also, integrating the additional information provided by the 31-GEP test with the American Joint Committee on Cancer (AJCC) online prognostic model (www.melanomaprognosis.net) significantly improved prognostic assessment.[52]

For SLNBx-negative patients, the 31-GEP test identified more than 80% of those patients who went on to develop distant metastases and expire. For patients with thin melanomas, a higher-risk 31-GEP result was more significantly associated with recurrence-free survival than SLNBx status.[53]

MANAGEMENT
Time to Surgery from Biopsy

It is known that early detection and treatment of melanoma leads to better outcomes. An analysis of time from biopsy to excisional surgery in patients with melanoma found that stage I patients who undergo surgery more than 30 days after biopsy have increased mortality risk.[54] Thus, it is integral to patient safety that excisional surgeries be performed as soon as reasonably feasible after biopsy.

Sentinel Lymph Node Biopsy

The guidelines for performing SLNBx remain in flux. The 2018 National Comprehensive Cancer Network (NCCN) guidelines recommend routine SLNBx for patients with a greater than 10% positivity rate.[55] They do not recommend this procedure in patients with a less than 5% rate of positive biopsy. For patients between 5% and 10%, discussion of the risks and benefits of the procedure with patients is recommended.

The American Society of Clinical Oncology (ASCO) also released updated guidelines for the management and staging of melanoma in 2018.[56]

- Thin melanomas: ASCO does not recommend routine SLNBx for patients with nonulcerated lesions less than 0.8 mm in thickness (stage T1a). Biopsy can be considered for melanomas 0.8 to 1.0 mm or less than 0.8 mm with ulceration (stage T1b).
- Intermediate-thickness melanomas: ASCO recommends SLNBx for melanomas that are 1.0 to 4 mm thick (stage T2 or T3).
- Thick melanomas: ASCO states that SLNBx may be recommended for patients with melanomas greater than 4 mm thick after thoroughly discussing benefits and risks of procedure.
- Completion lymph node dissection: ASCO recommends that either completion lymph node dissection or observation can be offered to patients with low risk of micrometastatic disease. For higher-risk patients, observation can be offered after a thorough discussion of potential risks and benefits of completion dissection.

Among patients with melanoma who undergo SLNBx, 84% are negative, suggesting that these patients do not benefit from the procedure.[57] For elderly patients, in whom positive SLNBx is rare, the 31-GEP test has a negative predictive value for SLNBx status of 96%.[58,59] With a less than 5% chance of positive SLNBx in this population, the 31-GEP test could potentially reduce the need for this invasive procedure.

Targeted Systemic Treatments

Four classes of targeted systemic treatments have been developed to treat melanoma (**Table 3**). The

Table 3
Pathways for targeted therapies in melanoma

Targeted Antitumor Therapy		Immune Checkpoint Blockade	
BRAF	*MEK*	*CTLA-4*	*PD-1*
Vemurafenib	Trametinib	Ipilimumab	Nivolumab
Dabrafenib	Cobimetinib	—	Pembrolizumab
—	—	—	Atezolizumab

BRAF inhibitors interrupt the B-raf/MEK step of the activation pathway. However, these drugs only work on melanomas with the B-raf V600E mutation. MEK inhibitors target the mitogen-activated protein kinase enzymes, MEK1 and/or MEK2. Phosphodiesterase-1 (PD-1) blockers halt PD-1's negative regulation of T cell effector mechanisms, which increases the T cell's ability to elicit an immune response against cancer. CTLA-4 antibodies block CTLA-4's ability to inhibit T cell responses.

The newest approaches to the treatment of advanced melanoma include combination therapy, an established mainstay of oncologic treatment in other types of cancers. Many combinations using drugs for different targets are being studied. A combination of BRAF and MEK inhibition in patients with V600E mutations found significantly increased survival among patients with combination therapy compared with monotherapy.[60] Similar results have been found in patients treated with a combination of a PD-1 blocker and CTLA-4 antibodies.[61] Triple combination therapies of a PD-1 blocker, BRAF inhibitor, and MEK inhibitor have also been successful in decreasing tumor burden.[62]

Dermatologic Side Effects of Targeted Therapies

Patients on BRAF inhibitors are more likely to develop de novo melanomas, squamous cell carcinomas, and keratoacanthomas during treatment because of activation of the *ras* pathway leading to BRAF-negative, ras-positive, newly appearing tumors.[63] The risk for developing these new melanomas is increased more than 1700 times in these patients compared with the general population. This fact reinforces the importance of close follow-up examination for patients on these drugs.

Patients on nivolumab frequently develop serious adverse events (11%) such as pneumonitis, vitiligo, colitis, hepatitis, hypophysitis, and thyroiditis.[64] In another study, cutaneous adverse events were seen in 49% of patients.[65]

PATIENT FOLLOW-UP

Patients who have been diagnosed with melanoma in situ or invasive melanoma have a 15 times increased lifetime risk of developing a subsequent primary melanoma, which equates to a 20% lifetime risk for being diagnosed with a second melanoma. Therefore, patients with melanoma need to be followed closely not only for the spread of disease from their initial tumors but also for the development of additional primary melanomas. A survey of dermatologists found that, within 5 years of melanoma diagnosis, most dermatologists follow their patients every 6 months.[66] After 5 years, the most common follow-up interval for dermatologists increased to yearly visits.

Cure for Melanoma?

Although a cure for melanoma does not currently exist, the possibility is clearly on the horizon. Survival intervals for patients with metastatic disease are increasing with the use of targeted approaches. Longer-term follow-up data from patients treated in the phase I study with the PD-1 blocker nivolumab showed that, for the one-third of patients who survived for 3 years on this therapy, almost all continued to survive at 7 years.[67]

SUMMARY

Approaches to melanoma diagnosis, management, and therapy are rapidly changing. Noninvasive devices and genetic testing can be used to help diagnose melanoma before a biopsy is done. Genetic expression profiling can help diagnose ambiguous melanomas and better predict patient outcomes. The advent of targeted systemic therapies has evolved metastatic melanoma from an automatic death sentence into one in which a small percentage of patients now have extended survivals. Despite these advances, the incidence of melanoma continues to increase, which reinforces the importance of a comprehensive understanding of all aspects of this cancer by dermatologists and the need for continued research to help make a material impact on this cancer.

REFERENCES

1. Siegel RL, Miller KD, Jemal A. Cancer statistics, 2018. CA Cancer J Clin 2018;68(1):7–30.
2. Siegel RL, Miller KD, Jemal A. Cancer statistics, 2017. CA Cancer J Clin 2017;67(1):7–30.
3. Erdmann F, Lortet-Tieulent J, Schüz J, et al. International trends in the incidence of malignant melanoma 1953-2008–are recent generations at higher or lower risk? Int J Cancer 2013;132(2):385–400.
4. American Cancer Society. Facts & figures 2018. Atlanta (GA): American Cancer Society; 2018.
5. Rastrelli M, Tropea S, Rossi CR, et al. Melanoma: epidemiology, risk factors, pathogenesis, diagnosis and classification. In Vivo 2014;28(6):1005–11.
6. Mitra D, Luo X, Morgan A, et al. An ultraviolet-radiation-independent pathway to melanoma carcinogenesis in the red hair/fair skin background. Nature 2012;491(7424):449–53.

7. Chen T, Fallah M, Kharazmi E, et al. Effect of a detailed family history of melanoma on risk for other tumors: a cohort study based on the nationwide Swedish Family-Cancer Database. J Invest Dermatol 2014;134(4):930–6.

8. Famenini S, Young LC. Aspirin use and melanoma risk: a review of the literature. J Am Acad Dermatol 2014;70:187–91.

9. Rachidi S, Wallace K, Li H, et al. Postdiagnosis aspirin use and overall survival in patients with melanoma. J Am Acad Dermatol 2018;78(5):949–56.e1.

10. Liu J, Shen B, Shi M, et al. Higher caffeinated coffee intake is associated with reduced malignant melanoma risk: a meta-analysis study. PLoS One 2016; 11(1):e0147056.

11. Wang J, Li X, Zhang D. Coffee consumption and the risk of cutaneous melanoma: a meta-analysis. Eur J Nutr 2016;55(4):1317–29.

12. Singh S, Nagpal SJ, Murad MH, et al. Inflammatory bowel disease is associated with an increased risk of melanoma: a systematic review and meta-analysis. Clin Gastroenterol Hepatol 2014;12(2):210–8.

13. Tang H, Wu W, Fu S, et al. Phosphodiesterase type 5 inhibitors and risk of melanoma: a meta-analysis. J Am Acad Dermatol 2017;77(3):480–8.e9.

14. Tellez A, Rueda S, Conic RZ, et al. Risk factors and outcomes of cutaneous melanoma in women less than 50 years of age. J Am Acad Dermatol 2016; 74(4):731–8.

15. Van der pols JC, Russell A, Bauer U, et al. Vitamin D status and skin cancer risk independent of time outdoors: 11-year prospective study in an Australian community. J Invest Dermatol 2013;133(3): 637–41.

16. Ally MS, Swetter SM, Hirotsu KE, et al. Promoting sunscreen use and sun-protective practices in NCAA athletes: impact of SUNSPORT educational intervention for student-athletes, athletic trainers, and coaches. J Am Acad Dermatol 2018;78(2): 289–92.e2.

17. Rzepecki AK, Jain N, Ali Y, et al. Promoting early detection of melanoma during the mammography experience. Int J Womens Dermatol 2017;3(4): 195–200.

18. Wu YP, Aspinwall LG, Conn BM, et al. A systematic review of interventions to improve adherence to melanoma preventive behaviors for individuals at elevated risk. Prev Med 2016;88:153–67.

19. American Academy of Dermatology. Check your partner infographic. Available at: https://www.aad.org/public/spot-skin-cancer/learn-about-skin-cancer/detect/check-your-partner-check-yourself. Accessed September 11, 2018.

20. Robinson JK, Wayne JD, Martini MC, et al. Early detection of new melanomas by patients with melanoma and their partners using a structured skin self-examination skills training intervention: a randomized clinical trial. JAMA Dermatol 2016; 152(9):979–85.

21. Green AC, Williams GM, Logan V, et al. Reduced melanoma after regular sunscreen use: randomized trial follow-up. J Clin Oncol 2011;29(3):257–63.

22. Olsen CM, Wilson LF, Green AC, et al. Cancers in Australia attributable to exposure to solar ultraviolet radiation and prevented by regular sunscreen use. Aust N Z J Public Health 2015;39(5):471–6.

23. Williams JD, Maitra P, Atillasoy E, et al. SPF 100+ sunscreen is more protective against sunburn than SPF 50+ in actual use: results of a randomized, double-blind, split-face, natural sunlight exposure clinical trial. J Am Acad Dermatol 2018;78(5): 902–10.

24. Mirsky RS, Prado G, Svoboda RM, et al. Oxybenzone and sunscreens: a critical review of the evidence and a plan for discussion with patients. Skin – J Cutan Med 2018;2(5):264–8.

25. Farrar MD, Huq R, Mason S, et al. Oral green tea catechins do not provide photoprotection from direct DNA damage induced by higher dose solar simulated radiation: a randomized controlled trial. J Am Acad Dermatol 2018;78(2):414–6.

26. Prado G, Winkelmann R, Del Rosso JQ, et al. Clinical efficacy & safety of oral polypodium leucotomos extract for photoprotection: a systematic review. American Academy of Dermatology Annual Meeting. Washington, DC, March 2, 2019. [abstract].

27. Vestergaard ME, Macaskill P, Holt PE, et al. Dermoscopy compared with naked eye examination for the diagnosis of primary melanoma: a meta-analysis of studies performed in a clinical setting. Br J Dermatol 2008;159(3):669–76.

28. Malvehy J, Hauschild A, Curiel-lewandrowski C, et al. Clinical performance of the Nevisense system in cutaneous melanoma detection: an international, multicentre, prospective and blinded clinical trial on efficacy and safety. Br J Dermatol 2014;171(5): 1099–107.

29. Bard RL. High frequency ultrasound examination in the diagnosis of skin cancer. Dermatol Clin 2017; 35(4):505–11.

30. Gerger A, Wiltgen M, Langsenlehner U, et al. Diagnostic image analysis of malignant melanoma in in vivo confocal laser-scanning microscopy: a preliminary study. Skin Res Technol 2008;14(3):359–63.

31. Gerami P, Yao Z, Polsky D, et al. Development and validation of a noninvasive 2-gene molecular assay for cutaneous melanoma. J Am Acad Dermatol 2017;76(1):114–20.e2.

32. Ferris LK, Gerami P, Skelsey MK, et al. Real-world performance and utility of a noninvasive gene expression assay to evaluate melanoma risk in pigmented lesions. Melanoma Res 2018;28(5):478–82.

33. Clarke LE, Warf MB, Flake DD, et al. Clinical validation of a gene expression signature that

differentiates benign nevi from malignant melanoma. J Cutan Pathol 2015;42(4):244–52.

34. Clarke LE, Flake DD, Busam K, et al. An independent validation of a gene expression signature to differentiate malignant melanoma from benign melanocytic nevi. Cancer 2017;123(4):617–28.

35. Ko JS, Matharoo-ball B, Billings SD, et al. Diagnostic distinction of malignant melanoma and benign nevi by a gene expression signature and correlation to clinical outcomes. Cancer Epidemiol Biomarkers Prev 2017;26(7):1107–13.

36. Cockerell CJ, Tschen J, Evans B, et al. The influence of a gene expression signature on the diagnosis and recommended treatment of melanocytic tumors by dermatopathologists. Medicine (Baltimore) 2016; 95(40):e4887.

37. Cockerell C, Tschen J, Billings SD, et al. The influence of a gene-expression signature on the treatment of diagnostically challenging melanocytic lesions. Per Med 2017;14(2):123–30.

38. Kooistra L, Chiang K, Dawes S, et al. Racial disparities and insurance status: an epidemiological analysis of Ohio melanoma patients. J Am Acad Dermatol 2018;78(5):998–1000.

39. Svoboda RM, Glazer AM, Farberg AS, et al. Melanoma reporting practices of United States dermatologists. Dermatol Surg 2018;44(11):1391–5.

40. Cartee TV, Kini SP, Chen SC. Melanoma reporting to central cancer registries by US dermatologists: an analysis of the persistent knowledge and practice gap. J Am Acad Dermatol 2011;65:S124–32.

41. Murtha TD, Han G, Han D. Predictors for use of sentinel node biopsy and the association with improved survival in melanoma patients who have nodal staging. Ann Surg Oncol 2018;25(4):903–11.

42. Morton DL, Thompson JF, Cochran AJ, et al. Final trial report of sentinel-node biopsy versus nodal observation in melanoma. N Engl J Med 2014; 370(7):599–609.

43. Sladden M, Zagarella S, Popescu C, et al. No survival benefit for patients with melanoma undergoing sentinel lymph node biopsy: critical appraisal of the Multicenter Selective Lymphadenectomy Trial-I final report. Br J Dermatol 2015;172(3):566–71.

44. Faries MB, Thompson JF, Cochran AJ, et al. Completion dissection or observation for sentinel-node metastasis in melanoma. N Engl J Med 2017; 376(23):2211–22.

45. Hsueh EC, Debloom JR, Lee J, et al. Interim analysis of survival in a prospective, multi-center registry cohort of cutaneous melanoma tested with a prognostic 31-gene expression profile test. J Hematol Oncol 2017;10(1):152.

46. Greenhaw BN, Zitelli JA, Brodland DG. Estimation of prognosis in invasive cutaneous melanoma: an independent study of the accuracy of a gene expression profile test. Dermatol Surg 2018;44(12):1494–500.

47. Zager JS, Gastman BR, Leachman S, et al. Performance of a prognostic 31-gene expression profile in an independent cohort of 523 cutaneous melanoma patients. BMC Cancer 2018;18(1):130.

48. Berger AC, Davidson RS, Poitras JK, et al. Clinical impact of a 31-gene expression profile test for cutaneous melanoma in 156 prospectively and consecutively tested patients. Curr Med Res Opin 2016; 32(9):1599–604.

49. Farberg AS, Glazer AM, White R, et al. Impact of a 31-gene expression profiling test for cutaneous melanoma on dermatologists' clinical management decisions. J Drugs Dermatol 2017;16(5):428–31.

50. Dillon LD, Gadzia JE, Davidson RS, et al. Prospective, multicenter clinical impact evaluation of a 31-gene expression profile test for management of melanoma patients. SKIN – J Cutan Med 2018; 2(2):111–21.

51. Gastman BR, Gerami P, Kurley SJ, et al. Identification of patients at risk for metastasis using a prognostic 31-gene expression profile 3 in subpopulations of melanoma patients with favorable outcomes by standard criteria. J Am Acad Dermatol 2019;80(1):149–57.e4.

52. Ferris LK, Farberg AS, Middlebrook B, et al. Identification of high-risk cutaneous melanoma tumors is improved when combining the online American Joint Committee on Cancer Individualized Melanoma Patient Outcome Prediction Tool with a 31-gene expression profile-based classification. J Am Acad Dermatol 2017;76(5):818–25.e3.

53. Cook RW, Covington KR, Monzon FA. Continued elevation of a 31-gene expression profile to predict metastasis in an expanded cohort of 782 cutaneous melanoma patients. Pigment Cell Res 2017;30(5): e73.

54. Conic RZ, Cabrera CI, Khorana AA, et al. Determination of the impact of melanoma surgical timing on survival using the National Cancer Database. J Am Acad Dermatol 2018;78(1):40–6.e7.

55. NCCN clinical practice guidelines in Oncology. Melanoma. Version 3. Available at: https://www.nccn.org/professionals/physician_gls/pdf/melanoma.pdf. Accessed September 12, 2018.

56. Wong SL, Faries MB, Kennedy EB, et al. Sentinel lymph node biopsy and management of regional lymph nodes in melanoma: American Society of Clinical Oncology and Society of Surgical Oncology clinical practice guideline update. J Clin Oncol 2018;36(4):399–413.

57. Morton DL, Thompson JF, Cochran AJ, et al. Sentinel-node biopsy or nodal observation in melanoma. N Engl J Med 2006;355(13):1307–17.

58. Macdonald JB, Dueck AC, Gray RJ, et al. Malignant melanoma in the elderly: different regional disease and poorer prognosis. J Cancer 2011;2: 538–43.

59. Vetto JT, Monzon FA, Cook RW, et al. Clinical utility of a 31-gene expression profile test to determine eligibility for sentinel lymph node biopsy in melanoma patients >65 years of age. American Academy of Dermatology Annual Meeting 2018. San Diego, CA, February 16, 2018.

60. Flaherty KT, Infante JR, Daud A, et al. Combined BRAF and MEK inhibition in melanoma with BRAF V600 mutations. N Engl J Med 2012;367(18): 1694–703.

61. Wolchok JD, Kluger H, Callahan MK, et al. Nivolumab plus ipilimumab in advanced melanoma. N Engl J Med 2013;369(2):122–33.

62. Ribas A, Hodi FS, Lawrence DP, et al. Pembrolizumab (pembro) in combination with dabrafenib (D) and trametinib (T) for *BRAF*-mutant advanced melanoma: Phase 1 KEYNOTE-022 study. J Clin Oncol 2016;34(15_suppl) [abstract: 3014].

63. Sosman JA, Kim KB, Schuchter L, et al. Survival in BRAF V600-mutant advanced melanoma treated with vemurafenib. N Engl J Med 2012;366(8): 707–14.

64. Topalian SL, Hodi FS, Brahmer JR, et al. Safety, activity, and immune correlates of anti-PD-1 antibody in cancer. N Engl J Med 2012;366(26):2443–54.

65. Hwang SJ, Carlos G, Wakade D, et al. Cutaneous adverse events (AEs) of anti-programmed cell death (PD)-1 therapy in patients with metastatic melanoma: a single-institution cohort. J Am Acad Dermatol 2016;74(3):455–61.e1.

66. Farberg AS, Rigel DS. A comparison of current practice patterns of US dermatologists versus published guidelines for the biopsy, initial management, and follow up of patients with primary cutaneous melanoma. J Am Acad Dermatol 2016;75(6):1193–7.e1.

67. Hodi FS, Kluger H, Sznol M, et al. Durable, long-term survival in previously treated patients with advanced melanoma (MEL) who received nivolumab (NIVO) monotherapy in a phase I trial. AACR 2016;76(14) [abstract: CT001].

Current Trends in Social Media–Associated Skin Harm Among Children and Adolescents

Albert C. Yan, MD[a,b,*]

KEYWORDS

- Social media • children • Adolescence • Self-injury • Pediatric • Challenge

KEY POINTS

- Tweens and teens may engage in self-injurious activities popularized by online social medial platforms that cause unintentional skin harm.
- Popular social media challenges include the eraser challenge, the salt-ice challenge, the deodorant challenge, and the fire challenge.
- These social media challenges can result in burns, persistent skin discoloration, scarring, and infection. In severe cases, patients have died from their injuries.
- Stick-and-poke tattoos, as well as homemade slime, can cause unintended harm; stick-and-poke tattoos may spread infection, and homemade slime has been linked to outbreaks of irritant contact dermatitis.

INTRODUCTION

Childhood and adolescence share several important hallmarks: the notable immaturity in understanding the potential consequences of individual actions are joined with tendencies toward impulsivity and a prioritization of gaining social acceptance, and can lead children and teens to poor decision making.

This is perhaps nowhere better exemplified than by the explosion of trending social media phenomena, often referred to as so-called social media "challenges." The more popular among these include those centered around pencil erasers, salt and ice, spray deodorant, and fire. Each of these share features of intentional self-injury with the possibility of permanent skin changes, although generally without the intent to cause harm. Rather, these provide secondary gain by fostering social acceptance or notoriety within their peer groups through postings on social media, although on occasion, they may represent attempts at school avoidance.

Other more innocuous self-administered activities, stick-and-poke tattoos as well as homemade slime hand dermatitis, although not technically social media challenges, are also activities disseminated by social medial that can also result in unintended complications of skin harm.

The background history of these social media–associated activities is both fascinating and perplexing. For the clinician, adept recognition of the characteristic skin signs of these behaviors affords the opportunity to discuss them in the open and to educate patients and their parents about how to avoid potential for more serious harm.

Disclosure Statement: No relevant financial disclosures.
[a] Section of Dermatology, Children's Hospital of Philadelphia, 3401 Civic Center Boulevard, Suite 3334, Philadelphia, PA 19104, USA; [b] Pediatrics and Dermatology, Perelman School of Medicine at the University of Pennsylvania, Philadelphia, PA, USA
* 3401 Civic Center Boulevard, Suite 3334, Philadelphia, PA 19104.
E-mail address: yana@email.chop.edu

Dermatol Clin 37 (2019) 169–174
https://doi.org/10.1016/j.det.2018.12.006

SOCIAL MEDIA PHENOMENA
Eraser Challenge

How it presents
Linear or geometric erosions or scars, typically on the hands, forearms, or occasionally other accessible body sites (**Fig. 1**).

What it is
(Friction burn) Those affected describe using a pencil eraser to rub the skin repeatedly, often until the patient completes the singing of the entire alphabet.

Commentary
This practice has been reported anecdotally for decades. However, since 2012, social media has helped disseminate this practice among school-aged children who at times will compete with one another to see who can achieve the largest or most impressive area of skin injury.[1] Although most appear to suffer only transient mild friction injury, enthusiastic practitioners may develop permanent scarring and secondary skin infections. In 2015, one child in Sacramento, California, was reportedly hospitalized after suffering from a toxic shock syndrome attributed to group A streptococcal infection.[2] Although it appears that many who do so are often seeking notoriety with their peers on social media, DeKlotz and Krakowski[3] reported on a 9-year-old patient who did so for secondary gain, as she was able to miss school to attend doctor's appointments.

Salt-Ice Challenge

How it presents
Geometric-shaped areas (often square) of violaceous erythema, sometimes with blistering or overlying erosions healing with erythema, dyspigmentation, or scarring.

What is it
(Cold thermal injury) Salt is placed on the skin and then ice cubes or crushed ice is then applied over the salt; because salt depresses the melting point of ice, it stays frozen for longer against the skin and is kept on for as long as the patient can tolerate (**Fig. 2**).

Commentary
This practice results in acute cold injury in the form of localized frostbite. In 2013, Williams and colleagues[4] described a 19-year-old young man who presented with 3 discrete geometric (rectangular) areas of frostbite on the forearm after succumbing to peer pressure while under the influence of alcohol. Preteens and teens have reported this as an initiation trial on sports teams, played as a game among friends competing against one another, or done to one another as a test of willpower. The degree of sequelae is related to the contact time, and although most will suffer only mild frostbite burns, more severe and extensive skin injury has been reported when some patients have undergone this challenge especially while under the influence of alcohol.[5]

Deodorant Challenge

How it presents
Solitary or multiple discrete, circular areas of violaceous erythema or blistering, resolving into areas of hyperpigmentation (**Fig. 3**)

What is it
(Cold thermal injury) Using a spray deodorant can, the aerosol is applied to an exposed area of the arm or leg. Patients reportedly enjoy watching the skin frost from the cooling effect of the aerosol. This activity produces a cold or frostbite injury with subsequent postinflammatory hyperpigmentation.[6]

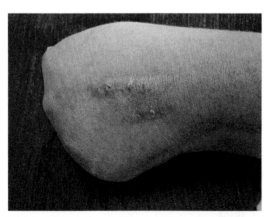

Fig. 1. Friction burn from eraser rubbed against the skin. (*Courtesy of* Andrew Krakowski, MD, Bethlehem, PA.)

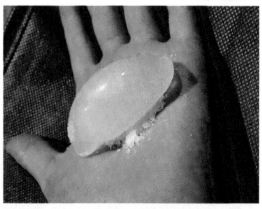

Fig. 2. Ice cube on bed of salt against the skin as part of the salt-ice challenge in a 10-year-old girl. (*Courtesy of* Albert Yan, MD, Philadelphia, PA.)

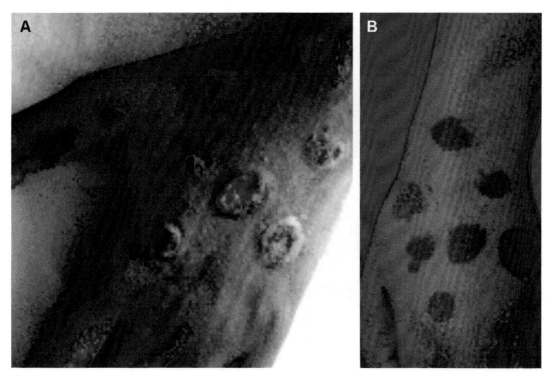

Fig. 3. (*A*) Multifocal areas of eroded skin caused by burns from sprayed aerosol deodorant. (*B*) Multifocal areas of residual hyperpigmentation following healing of deodorant burns. (*Reproduced from* Soysal N, Bourrat E. The deodorant game: a diagnostic challenge in paediatric dermatology. Ann Dermatol Venereol 2017;144(5):384–6.

Commentary

Aerosol-induced cold injury is a known mechanism for intentional self-injury among adolescents. Traditionally, this has been produced using beta-agonist inhalers and represents one of the most common sources of chemical burns in children.[7] More recently, children have been using spray deodorants, which can produce more intense cold injury, using this as a test of willpower to see how long they can tolerate the spraying. Localized blistering can occur, followed by prolonged hyperpigmentation and occasionally scarring at the affected sites.[8]

Fire Challenge

How it presents

Irregular areas of erythema and skin denudation at sites of thermal burns, healing with dyschromia and scarring.

What is it

(Thermal burn) Patients report using perfume or rubbing alcohol as an accelerant, and either spray it on themselves or onto a friend before setting it on fire using a lighter or match.[9]

Commentary

The fire challenge poses perhaps the greatest risk to those who do it because of the potential for unanticipated uncontrolled spread of the flames. Patients who have done this often report after the fact that they had no idea that the fire would burn them, a misunderstanding borne of seeing the stunt posted on social media by survivors of the challenge and misconceptions that fire arising from burning of alcohol can still burn the skin. Although some teens are clever enough to perform this in a shower and run the shower immediately after lighting to douse the fire, others have not been so fortunate, and there have been incidents of second-degree and third-degree burns requiring grafting, with resulting dyschromia and scarring.[9] Unfortunately, fatalities also have been reported in association with this practice.[10] Notably, a disproportion of patients affected have been young African American male individuals, suggesting that this population may be at special risk and warrant greater attention for education efforts.[9]

Stick-and-Poke Tattoos

How it presents

Permanent tattoos, often using black ink (**Fig. 4**). Most are simple, although professional tattoo artists can use this same technique to produce complex artwork in the skin.

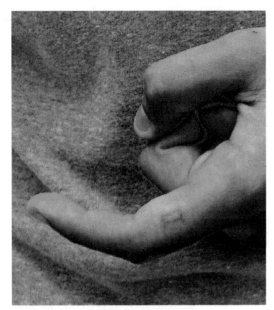

Fig. 4. Stick-and-poke tattoo obtained at a birthday party. (*Courtesy of* Albert Yan, MD, Philadelphia, PA.)

What is it

(Tattoo) Tattoo parties have emerged as a birthday party theme among young people. Most commonly, this involves the application of ballpoint ink and stick pins or sewing needles to instill ink into the skin in the desired pattern.

Commentary

This practice derives from long-standing, inexpensive, tattooing traditions. However, patients are often under the mistaken impression that these tattoos are temporary, and only find out to their later regret that these are permanent. Fortunately, they can be removed with laser. However, because of the lack of hygienic practices associated with this, including the sharing of needles and pins, patients put themselves at risk for secondary infection with viruses, bacteria, and fungi. Reports of stick-and-poke tattooing resulting in infection are plentiful on social media. Several documented cases of significant secondary infections following stick-and-poke tattoos have been reported, including deep fungal infection from aspergillus.[11]

Slime Dermatitis

How it presents

Well-demarcated areas of glossy erythema involving the palms (**Fig. 5**).

What it is

(Irritant contact dermatitis) Children's play slime is a compound created from a mixture of water, polyvinyl acetate glue, such as Elmer's, and sodium borate.[12] The resulting compound is often mixed

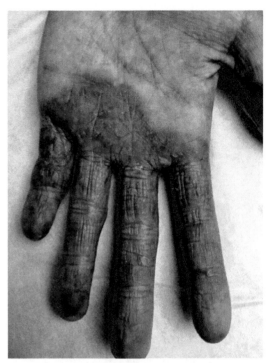

Fig. 5. Slime contact dermatitis of the palms. (*Courtesy of* Leonard Kristal, MD, Stony Brook, NY.)

with food coloring, glitter, and confetti. Children often make their own slime at home and may spend hours a day playing with it using their hands to knead it.

Commentary

Making slime has become a popular activity among children as an arts and crafts project in

Table 1 Pervasiveness of social media–associated phenomena			
Social Media Phenomenon	Origin Date	Videos on YouTube (as of July 2018)	Hits on Google (as of September 2018)
Stick-and-poke tattoos	2008	28,000	12,700,000
Salt-ice challenge	2012	830,000	54,100,000
Eraser challenge	2013	313,000	8,540,000
Fire challenge	2014	12,300,000	421,000,000
Deodorant challenge	2017	127,000	7,900,000
Slime burns	2017	6550	3,860,000

Table 2
Contrasting features of child abuse, nonsuicidal self-injury, and social media–associated skin harm

	Child Abuse	Nonsuicidal Self-Injury (DSM-5)	Social Media–Associated Skin Harm
Patterned skin injury	Yes	Yes	Yes
Occasional or repetitive instances	Repetitive	Either	Either
Intent to harm	Yes	Yes	No
Underlying psychopathology	Yes (abuser)	No (for occasional) Yes (for repetitive)	No
Intent	Performed to dole out punishment	Often associated with antecedent negative emotional states	Performed out of curiosity or desire to gain acceptance or notoriety within social group

DSM-5, diagnostic and statistical manual of mental disorders, fifth edition.

schools or at home. Parents often have no objection to having their children use science to transform ingredients into a popular toy, but reports have emerged in the lay press as well as in social media of chemical burns or significant irritant contact dermatitis resulting from prolonged skin exposure to play slime, and several reports have highlighted this phenomenon in the medical literature.[13–15] A subset of cases may also be linked to allergic contact dermatitis, with one case directly linked to sensitization to methylisothiazolinone.[16]

SUMMARY

Although there are many benefits to social media, these platforms have also emerged as a means of popularizing a number of questionable practices that can produce skin harm. These are forms of nonaccidental trauma that are typically intentional, self-induced, and performed for secondary gain: namely, for the purposes of gaining social acceptance or notoriety or occasionally for school avoidance. These phenomena carry significant risk for cutaneous complications, including but not limited to pain, discomfort, dyschromia, scarring, and secondary infection.

Unfortunately, social media has proven an effective means of permitting the widespread dissemination of these practices, and has allowed young people the opportunity to learn about these and to act on them. As of this writing, thousands of videos are accessible on YouTube, and there are millions of hits on search engines such as Google (**Table 1**). The sheer volume of available content can mask the potential morbidity and occasional mortality that can arise in association with these activities.

The differential diagnosis of patterned skin injury includes nonaccidental trauma arising from child abuse. This is typically perpetrated on the child by a caregiver and results in patterned skin injury, and there is often a discordance between the skin manifestations and the history provided. Nonsuicidal self-injury disorder has recently been included as a diagnosis in the *Diagnostic and Statistical Manual of Mental Disorders* (5th Edition)[17] and is characterized by either occasional or repetitive self-injury for purposes of self-injury that are not socially sanctioned, and includes cutting, scratching, biting, or burning. This type of behavior can be triggered by negative feelings or stressful events. In some cases, underlying psychopathology, such as borderline personality disorder, can be associated.[18] It should also be remembered that patterned intentional skin injury also may result from cultural healing practices, such as cupping or coining.

It is important for clinicians to recognize related skin manifestations (**Table 2**), and be capable and ready to distinguish them from skin signs of child abuse or intentional self-injury as a feature of an underlying psychiatric disorder.

REFERENCES

1. Available at: https://www.today.com/health/eraser-challenge-what-parents-need-know-about-craze-t109100. Accessed September 26, 2018.
2. Available at: https://www.wnd.com/2015/10/teen-hospitalized-after-eraser-challenge-game/. Accessed September 26, 2018.
3. DeKlotz CM, Krakowski AC. The eraser challenge among school-age children. J Clin Aesthet Dermatol 2013;6(12):45–6.
4. Williams JMD, Cubitt JJ, Dickson WA. The challenge of salt and ice. Burns 2013;39:1024–30.
5. Available at: https://www.cbsnews.com/news/ice-and-salt-challenge-leaves-12-year-old-pittsburgh-boy-

with-second-degree-burns/. Accessed September 26, 2018.

6. Soysal N, Bourrat E. The deodorant game: a diagnostic challenge in paediatric dermatology. Ann Dermatol Venereol 2017;144(5):384–6.

7. D'Cruz R, Pang TC, Harvey JG, et al. Chemical burns in children: aetiology and prevention. Burns 2015;41(4):764–9.

8. Available at: http://time.com/5270672/deodorant-challenge-trend-burns-warning/. Accessed September 24, 2018.

9. Avery AH, Rae L, Sumitt JB, et al. The fire challenge: a case report and analysis of self-inflicted flame injury posted on social media. J Burn Care Res 2016;37(2):e161–5.

10. Available at: https://www.news965.com/news/local/facebook-fire-challenge-goes-horribly-wrong/1zaeYrTOK3cw6MTkmJ5wUJ/. Accessed September 26, 2018.

11. Kluger N, Saarinen K. *Aspergillus fumigatus* infection on a home-made tattoo. Br J Dermatol 2014;170(6):1373–5.

12. Available at: https://www.wikihow.com/Make-Slime-with-Borax. Accessed September 26, 2018.

13. Heller E, Murthy AS, Jen MV. A slime of the times: two cases of acute irritant contact dermatitis from homemade slime. Pediatr Dermatol 2018. https://doi.org/10.1111/pde.13617.

14. Aerts O, DeFre C, van Hoof T, et al. "Slime": a new fashion among children causing severe hand dermatitis. Contact Dermatitis 2018. https://doi.org/10.1111/cod.13090.

15. Gittler JK, Garzon MC, Lauren CT. "Slime" may not be so benign: a cause of hand dermatitis. J Pediatr 2018;200:288.

16. Zhang AJ, Boyd AH, Asch S, et al. Allergic contact dermatitis to slime: The epidemic of isothiazolinone encompasses school glue. Pediatric Dermatology 2019;36(1):e37–8.

17. American Psychiatric Association. Diagnostic and statistical manual of mental disorders. 5th edition. Arlington, VA: American Psychiatric Association; 2013.

18. Zetterqvist M. The DSM-5 diagnosis of nonsuicidal self-injury disorder: a review of the empirical literature. Child Adolesc Psychiatry Ment Health 2015;9(31). https://doi.org/10.1186/s13034-015-0062-7.

What's New in Pigmentary Disorders

Raheel Zubair, MD, MHS[a], Alexis B. Lyons, MD[a], Gautham Vellaichamy, BS[a,b], Anjelica Peacock, BS[b], Iltefat Hamzavi, MD[a,*]

KEYWORDS

- Pigmentary disorders • Vitiligo • Melasma • Management • Postinflammatory hyperpigmentation

KEY POINTS

- Pigmentary disorders encompass a multitude of diseases with many areas of ongoing research.
- There are several promising new treatments for vitiligo with burgeoning evidence, including melanocyte-keratinocyte transplant procedure, afamelanotide, and Janus kinase inhibitors.
- The risk of postinflammatory hyperpigmentation must be taken into consideration when using lasers to treat any form of hyperpigmentation.
- Fractional and picosecond lasers, as well as the use of low fluence, large spot size settings, may decrease this risk.

INTRODUCTION

Pigmentary disorders include both hypopigmentation and hyperpigmentation. The most common pigmentary disorders are typically not life threatening or associated with health risks; however, they can have substantial negative effects on emotional well-being and quality of life. These effects can also be exacerbated by stigmatization. Pigmentary disorders may also disproportionately affect people with skin of color.[1] Although pigmentary disorders are relatively common, they remain challenging to treat. This article reviews emerging therapies for some of these more common disorders. These therapies encompass a wide range of modalities including topicals, systemic agents, light treatments, and lasers. This information can help clinicians to expand their toolkit when facing pigmentary disorders.

VITILIGO

Vitiligo is a disorder characterized by white macules and patches resulting from the loss of functional melanocytes. Although it is common, there remain no completely satisfactory treatments. Currently accepted treatment options include topical steroids, calcineurin inhibitors, and narrow-band UVB phototherapy, but these modalities have had varied rates of success. There are newer, experimental treatments that show some promise.

Afamelanotide

Afamelanotide is a linear analogue of α-melanocyte-stimulating hormone, an endogenous peptide that stimulates melanocyte proliferation and melanogenesis.[2] Afamelanotide is also called melanotan I, and is marketed under the trade name SCENESSE by Clinuvel (Melbourne, Australia). Melanotan II is another synthetic form of α-melanocyte-stimulating hormone with a shortened, circular configuration. Both melanotan I and II result in sunless tanning but commonly cause nausea; melanotan II also causes increased libido and spontaneous erections.

A 2015 randomized multicenter trial of adults with nonsegmental vitiligo in skin types III to VI found that the combination of a subcutaneous

Disclosure: Dr A.B. Lyons, Dr R. Zubair, and Dr I. Hamzavi are investigators for The Estée Lauder Companies Inc., Incyte Corp and Unigen Corporation.

[a] Department of Dermatology, Henry Ford Hospital System, 3031 West Grand Boulvard, Suite 800, Detroit, MI 48202, USA; [b] Wayne State University School of Medicine, 540 East Canfield Street, Detroit, MI 48201, USA
* Corresponding author.
E-mail address: Iltefat@hamzavi.com

Dermatol Clin 37 (2019) 175–181
https://doi.org/10.1016/j.det.2018.12.008
0733-8635/19/© 2018 Elsevier Inc. All rights reserved.

afamelanotide implant and narrow band UVB phototherapy was superior to narrow band UVB monotherapy in producing repigmentation. The combination therapy group had 48.64% repigmentation at day 168 and the monotherapy narrow band UVB group had 33.26% repigmentation over the same time period.[2] For the most easily visible locations, including the face and upper extremities, the median time to onset of repigmentation was 20 days shorter in the combination therapy group. There was also a trend toward a quicker response in darker phototypes. The most common adverse events were erythema and hyperpigmentation; a majority of patients in both groups experienced erythema. Hyperpigmentation of unaffected skin was experienced by all members of the combination therapy group, and 2 patients were bothered by this effect enough to withdraw from the study. Future studies are needed to investigate the efficacy of afamelanotide in fair-skinned patients as well as its use as a monotherapy.

Melanocyte–Keratinocyte Transplant Procedure and Noncultured Epidermal Suspension Surgery

Melanocyte–keratinocyte transplantation is a surgery for patients with vitiligo and was first described by Gauthier and Surleve-Bazeille in 1992.[3] In this procedure, epidermal cells are harvested from a donor site and grafted as a suspension, which allows for the treatment of a recipient site 10 times larger than the donor area.[4] Patients with stable segmental vitiligo and without a history of koebnerization, hypertrophic scarring, keloids, or poor wound healing are good candidates. Patients with fingertip and periorificial involvement are excluded, because they are unlikely to repigment in response to melanocyte–keratinocyte transplantation.[4] The proximal, lateral thigh is often used as a donor site, because it is flat and cosmetically acceptable. After local and/or topical anesthesia is used, ultrathin (<0.125 mm) skin grafts are harvested using either a Silvers skin grafting knife or a sterile razor held with hemostats. The graft is then incubated in trypsin. Forceps are used to separate the dermis, which is discarded, from the epidermis. The epidermis is divided into small fragments and centrifuged to create a cell pellet that will be resuspended. While the suspension is being prepared, the recipient site is anesthetized and made denuded by either fractional CO_2 laser ablation or dermabrasion. At this point, the suspension is applied through the hub of a needleless syringe and the wound is dressed using collagen matrix and gauze. Repigmentation begins 2 to 8 weeks after surgery and full pigmentation is achieved within 6 to 18 months. A study of 23 patients who underwent melanocyte–keratinocyte transplantation evaluated repigmentation at treatment sites and found that 17% were graded as excellent (95%–100% repigmentation), 31% were good (65%–94%), 10% were fair (25%–64%), and 41% were poor (0%–24%).[5] The mean improvement in the Vitiligo Area Scoring Index was 45%.

Melanocyte–keratinocyte transplantation is continually being improved and simplified. The donor skin harvesting procedure may be streamlined by a new automated epidermal harvesting system that uses negative pressure to create suction blisters, which are used as epidermal micrografts.[6] Melanocyte–keratinocyte transplantation is safe and effective, but it is not widely performed for several reasons: There are only a few practitioners who are trained to perform the procedure, it is not widely known among patients or physicians, and there is a lack of payer support, resulting in high out-of-pocket costs.

Bimatoprost

Bimatoprost is a synthetic prostaglandin analogue.[7,8] Currently, this drug is used as an ophthalmic solution for glaucoma to decrease intraocular pressure by increasing aqueous outflow and to treat eyelash hypotrichosis.[7,9] It has been shown that bimatoprost also induces periocular hyperpigmentation caused by increased melanogenesis without proliferation of melanocytes or prostaglandin-induced inflammation.[10] Further research has shown increased skin pigmentation in all areas with the use of bimatoprost, latanoprost, and travoprost combined with and without narrow band UVB therapy in adult female guinea pigs.[11] With this information, studies have been conducted to determine the efficacy of bimatoprost as a vitiligo treatment.

Jha and colleagues[12,13] have reported bimatoprost ophthalmic solution causing repigmentation in periorbital vitiligo and eyebrow leukotrichia. The same authors also reported a series of 8 cases of stable facial vitiligo treated with bimatoprost 0.03% ophthalmic solution daily for 12 weeks.[14] Repigmentation was graded as excellent (75%–100%) in 4 cases, partial (25%–50%) in 2 cases, and poor (<25%) in 2 cases.[14] Grimes[15] conducted a randomized, double-blind clinical trial to assess bimatoprost's ability to repigment skin in nonfacial vitiligo. Their group recruited 32 subjects with nonfacial vitiligo and divided them into 3 arms: bimatoprost monotherapy, bimatoprost with mometasone, and mometasone with placebo. This study showed that bimatoprost, both as a monotherapy and in combination with mometasone, is more effective than mometasone alone in the treatment of nonfacial vitiligo.[15]

Although these treatments are promising, there are limitations to this particular drug particularly when applied intraocularly. Changes in iris pigmentation have been associated with bimatoprost when administered as an eye drop for glaucoma treatment.[16] Other reported side effects include conjunctival hyperemia, pruritus, burning sensation in the eye, eye pain, eyelash growth, foreign body sensation, visual disturbances, and dryness.[17] As mentioned elsewhere in this article, larger scale studies need to be conducted to assess the safety and efficacy in bimatoprost in the treatment of vitiligo.

Janus Kinase Inhibitors

Janus kinase inhibitors (JAK inhibitors) are an emerging treatment option that have shown significant potential in recent years for the treatment of pigmentary disorders, particularly those with an underlying autoimmune etiology, such as vitiligo. Mouse models have demonstrated that vitiligo has an IFN-γ–specific signature underlying its pathogenesis.[18] IFN-γ binds to JAK receptors, initiating secondary signaling via the JAK-STAT pathway and producing the chemokine CXCL10, which proceeds to bind to the CXCR3 receptor on CD8 cytotoxic T cells.[18] These CD8 T cells are then directed to destroy native melanocytes causing the phenotypic depigmentation characteristic of vitiligo.[18–20] Thus, by blocking the activation of the JAK-STAT pathway, JAK inhibitors stop production of CXCL10 and shut down this process.

Two JAK inhibitors, tofacitinib and ruxolitinib, are being actively investigated as treatments for vitiligo and other pigmentary disorders.[20] They are approved for other organ pathologies, including rheumatoid arthritis and myelofibrosis, and now have burst onto the dermatology scene.[21,22] Both drugs were introduced in separate case studies in which oral administration resulted in significant to complete repigmentation of vitiligo lesions and their discontinuation resulted in recurrence of depigmentation.[19,20,23] Additionally, a topical formulation of 1.5% ruxolitinib has shown efficacy in a 12-patient, 20-week, open-label study.[24] A 32-week extension of this study with the same methodology showed a statistically significant mean improvement in the overall Vitiligo Area Scoring Index score at week 52.[25] A retrospective case series also suggests that there is a synergistic effect with low-level light, so JAK inhibitors may become an adjunct to phototherapy for

pigmentary disorders.[26] JAK inhibitors are generally deemed to be safe.[20] Other dermatologic disease that often genetically coexist with vitiligo such as alopecia areata have responded to ruxolitinib and tofacitinib therapy, albeit only in the oral form.[23] Although JAK inhibitors hold great potential, there remain knowledge gaps regarding the dosing and safety profile.[27]

MELASMA

Melasma is a common, chronic disorder thought to be the result of UV exposure and hormonal contributions resulting in hyperpigmented macules and patches on the face. Despite its common occurrence, there is no cure, and it remains difficult to treat. The best treatment approaches depend on whether the location of the pigment is epidermal, dermal, or both.

Photoprotection

Photoprotection is of the utmost importance in controlling melasma. It has now been established that not only UV light, but also visible light can induce sustained dark pigmentation in darker skinned patients.[28] The implication of this fact for patients is that they should use sunscreens with physical agents, such as titanium dioxide and zinc oxide, rather than chemical agents, which are not effective against visible light.

Hydroquinone

Hydroquinone (HQ) is a first-line treatment for melasma and is the most commonly used depigmentation agent. Its mechanism of action is the competitive inhibition of tyrosinase, the enzyme responsible for melanin synthesis. Rarely, prolonged use of HQ at high concentration can result exogenous ochronosis by causing an accumulation of homogentisic acid. An 8-week trial found that a triple combination cream of HQ 4%, tretinoin 0.05%, and fluocinolone acetonide 0.01% was significantly more effective than HQ 4% alone.[29] Both groups had similar incidence of erythema, desquamation, and burning sensations. The inclusion of a steroid, however, makes this combination problematic for maintenance therapy of melasma because it may cause steroid-induced atrophy.

Kojic Acid

Another emerging treatment for melasma is kojic acid. Kojic acid chelates the copper in tyrosinase and is produced by *Aspergillus* fungi. In a 12-week trial of 60 subjects in India comparing HQ 4.00% with 0.75% kojic acid cream, HQ was superior to kojic acid at improving melasma as measured by the Melasma Area and Severity Index (MASI).[30] Another-12 week Indian study of 80 patients compared the efficacy of kojic acid 1% alone and in various combinations with HQ 2% and betamethasone valerate 0.1%. The greatest improvement in MASI score was found in the group that received kojic acid in combination with HQ.[31]

Tranexamic Acid

Oral tranexamic acid (TXA) has shown to be a promising treatment for treatment-resistant melasma.[32] It is the first systemic therapy for melasma, was first described as a potential therapy in 1979, and demonstrated improvement after 4 weeks of treatment.[33] Since then, many studies have tested oral TXA in Asian populations with good results and no serious side effects.[34–40] More recently, a randomized, placebo-controlled, double-blind study of oral TXA on primarily Hispanic white women showed a greater decrease in modified MASI in the oral TXA group (49% reduction) when compared with the placebo group (18% decrease) with no serious adverse events.[41] Its effect on melasma is thought to work through several mechanisms, including the inhibition of epidermal melanocyte tyrosinase activity, preventing the binding of plasminogen to keratinocytes, and decreasing levels of α-melanocyte-stimulating hormone.[42] Patients should be screened before treatment with oral TXA, but of the studies discussed, none showed a significant risk for thrombosis in the healthy general population unless an underlying clotting disorder or risk factor was present.

Fractional Q-Switched Ruby Laser

The use of lasers for melasma treatment has had mixed results and is associated with hypopigmentation and postinflammatory hyperpigmentation (PIH). Q-switched ruby lasers (QSRL) are no exception to this trend. Multiple trials have had mixed results—subjects developed PIH, did not have long-term improvement, and sometimes had worsening of their melasma.[43,44] Somewhat better results have been achieved with fractional QSRL. Fractional lasers deliver the beam as an array of microthermal treatment zones. There are intervening untreated areas between these zones that enable faster healing between treatments. This provides a theoretic basis for why fractional QSRL may minimize PIH compared with classical QSRL. In 25 Caucasian patients, Hilton and colleagues[45] observed a 72.3% reduction in MASI score at 4 to 6 follow-up after a mean of 1.4 laser treatments of 4 to 8 J/cm^2. After 3 months, PIH

was observed in 7 patients and recurrent melasma was observed in 11 patients. Jang and colleagues[46] used 6 treatments at a lower fluence of 2 to 3 J/cm^2 at 2-week intervals and were able to achieve a 30% improvement in MASI score. Pain and erythema were minimal in both studies. Neither group followed patients for more than 4 months, so longer term studies are needed.

Q-Switched Nd:YAG Laser

The long wavelength of 1064 nm Nd:YAG allows it to penetrate deeply, better treat dermal and mixed pigmentation, and minimize the risk of PIH. There are also frequency doubled 532 nm Nd:YAG lasers that may be more effective for epidermal melasma. There have several trials testing the idea of laser toning to treat melasma by using multiple pass of QS Nd:YAG at low fluence (1–4 J/cm^2) with large spot size (6–10 mm). Sixteen patients of skin types I to IV with moderate mixed-type melasma were given 6 treatments at 1-week intervals of low fluence 1064 nm QS Nd:YAG.[47] Moderate improvement of MASI score was observed, and other small trials have had similar results.[48,49] Wattanakrai and colleagues[50] used comparable laser treatments on 22 Asian patients, but found that improvements were temporary and rebound hyperpigmentation and mottled hypopigmentation were common. All patients had recurrent melasma.

Picosecond Laser

Another emerging mode of treatment for melasma is the picosecond laser. The use of this type of laser with such a short pulse duration allows for reduction in the photothermal effect generated during removal of pigment and therefore less damage to the surrounding normal tissue.[51] It has been shown to be superior when used in combination with HQ when compared with HQ alone.[52,53] Further studies are needed to elucidate the ideal settings and treatment parameters for the various Fitzpatrick skin types.

POSTINFLAMMATORY HYPERPIGMENTATION

PIH is a hypermelanosis reaction to inflammation. It occurs more frequently in patients with darker skin. PIH may be caused by endogenous dermatoses, such as acne, or external injury. The inciting source of inflammation should be controlled first to prevent PIH from developing or worsening.

Treatment of existing PIH has some overlap with melasma. For example, HQ is a first-line treatment, whereas other depigmenting agents and laser therapies are second line. The use of lasers for

PIH is controversial, because it is not only refractory to laser therapy, but PIH is also not an uncommon side effect of laser therapies in general. Taylor and Anderson[43] found the QSRL to be ineffective for PIH. Cho and colleagues[54] published a report of 3 Korean patients who underwent 5 treatments using 1064 nm QS Nd:YAG at low fluence, similar to the methods described for melasma. Their PIH remained improved 2 months after the final treatment. There are also case reports of fractional photothermolysis being used successfully to improve PIH.[55,56] In general, any laser treatment for PIH should be done very cautiously, especially in darker skin types. As with melasma, all patients should use photoprotection.

One obstacle to performing robust therapeutic studies was the lack of a validated scoring system for PIH. Savory and colleagues[57] developed the postacne hyperpigmentation index and evaluated its use on 21 patients. The postacne hyperpigmentation index had good interrater reliability and correlated well with quality-of-life scores. This instrument may help to standardize and facilitate comparison between PIH treatment studies.

SUMMARY

The field of pigmentary skin disorders is continually evolving with several innovative therapies emerging for each condition. In the future, the best combination of topical, systemic, and light treatments for each disorder will become better elucidated. Unfortunately, many of these conditions, despite the disfiguring and devastating effects on patient self-esteem and quality of life, are still considered cosmetic by health insurance and other payers. Although treatment options are improving, the lack of payer support, and the refractory, recurrent nature of these diseases make complete resolution quite challenging to achieve. Even among the most encouraging therapies, there remains a need for larger trials with extended follow-up times to establish the longevity of treatment results. Pigmentary abnormalities have long been a neglected area and patients have suffered. Progress is being made, but only through rigorous studies and patient advocacy can true advances be made.

REFERENCES

1. Taylor A, Pawaskar M, Taylor SL, et al. Prevalence of pigmentary disorders and their impact on quality of life: a prospective cohort study. J Cosmet Dermatol 2008;7(3):164–8.
2. Lim HW, Grimes PE, Agbai O, et al. Afamelanotide and narrowband UV-B phototherapy for the treatment of vitiligo: a randomized multicenter trial. JAMA Dermatol 2015;151(1):42–50.
3. Gauthier Y, Surleve-Bazeille J-E. Autologous grafting with noncultured melanocytes: a simplified method for treatment of depigmented lesions. J Am Acad Dermatol 1992;26(2):191–4.
4. Nahhas AF, Mohammad TF, Hamzavi IH. Vitiligo surgery: shuffling melanocytes. J Investig Dermatol Symp Proc 2017;18(2):S34–7.
5. Huggins RH, Henderson MD, Mulekar SV, et al. Melanocyte-keratinocyte transplantation procedure in the treatment of vitiligo: the experience of an academic medical center in the United States. J Am Acad Dermatol 2012;66(5):785–93.
6. Budania A, Parsad D, Kanwar A, et al. Comparison between autologous noncultured epidermal cell suspension and suction blister epidermal grafting in stable vitiligo: a randomized study. Br J Dermatol 2012;167(6):1295–301.
7. Woodward DF, Krauss AH, Chen J, et al. The pharmacology of bimatoprost (Lumigan). Surv Ophthalmol 2001;45(Suppl 4):S337–45.
8. Woodward DF, Liang Y, Krauss AH. Prostamides (prostaglandin-ethanolamides) and their pharmacology. Br J Pharmacol 2008;153(3):410–9.
9. Bagherani N, Smoller BR. Efficacy of bimatoprost in the treatment of non-facial vitiligo. Dermatol Ther 2017;30(2). https://doi.org/10.1111/dth.12409.
10. Kapur R, Osmanovic S, Toyran S, et al. Bimatoprost-induced periocular skin hyperpigmentation: histopathological study. Arch Ophthalmol 2005;123(11):1541–6.
11. Anbar TS, El-Ammawi TS, Barakat M, et al. Skin pigmentation after NB-UVB and three analogues of prostaglandin F(2alpha) in guinea pigs: a comparative study. J Eur Acad Dermatol Venereol 2010;24(1):28–31.
12. Jha AK, Sinha R, Prasad S, et al. Bimatoprost in periorbital vitiligo: a ray of hope or dilemma. J Eur Acad Dermatol Venereol 2016;30(7):1247–8.
13. Jha AK, Sinha R. Bimatoprost in vitiligo. Clin Exp Dermatol 2016;41(7):821–2.
14. Jha AK, Prasad S, Sinha R. Bimatoprost ophthalmic solution in facial vitiligo. J Cosmet Dermatol 2018;17(3):437–40.
15. Grimes PE. Bimatoprost 0.03% solution for the treatment of nonfacial vitiligo. J Drugs Dermatol 2016;15(6):703–10.
16. Williams RD, Cohen JS, Gross RL, et al. Long-term efficacy and safety of bimatoprost for intraocular pressure lowering in glaucoma and ocular hypertension: year 4. Br J Ophthalmol 2008;92(10):1387–92.
17. Higginbotham EJ, Schuman JS, Goldberg I, et al. One-year, randomized study comparing bimatoprost and timolol in glaucoma and ocular hypertension. Arch Ophthalmol 2002;120(10):1286–93.
18. Rashighi M, Agarwal P, Richmond JM, et al. CXCL10 is critical for the progression and maintenance of

depigmentation in a mouse model of vitiligo. Sci Transl Med 2014;6(223):223ra223.

19. Craiglow BG, King BA. Tofacitinib citrate for the treatment of vitiligo: a pathogenesis-directed therapy. JAMA Dermatol 2015;151(10):1110–2.

20. Damsky W, King BA. JAK inhibitors in dermatology: the promise of a new drug class. J Am Acad Dermatol 2017;76(4):736–44.

21. Zerbini CA, Lomonte AB. Tofacitinib for the treatment of rheumatoid arthritis. Expert Rev Clin Immunol 2012;8(4):319–31.

22. Mesa RA, Yasothan U, Kirkpatrick P. Ruxolitinib. Nat Rev Drug Discov 2012;11(2):103–4.

23. Harris JE, Rashighi M, Nguyen N, et al. Rapid skin repigmentation on oral ruxolitinib in a patient with coexistent vitiligo and alopecia areata (AA). J Am Acad Dermatol 2016;74(2):370–1.

24. Rothstein B, Joshipura D, Saraiya A, et al. Treatment of vitiligo with the topical Janus kinase inhibitor ruxolitinib. J Am Acad Dermatol 2017;76(6):1054–60.e1.

25. Joshipura D, Alomran A, Zancanaro P, et al. Treatment of vitiligo with the topical Janus kinase inhibitor ruxolitinib: a 32-week open-label extension study with optional narrow-band ultraviolet B. J Am Acad Dermatol 2018;78(6):1205–7.e1.

26. Liu LY, Strassner JP, Refat MA, et al. Repigmentation in vitiligo using the Janus kinase inhibitor tofacitinib may require concomitant light exposure. J Am Acad Dermatol 2017;77(4):675–82.e1.

27. Shreberk-Hassidim R, Ramot Y, Zlotogorski A. Janus kinase inhibitors in dermatology: a systematic review. J Am Acad Dermatol 2017;76(4):745–53.e19.

28. Mahmoud BH, Ruvolo E, Hexsel CL, et al. Impact of long-wavelength UVA and visible light on melanocompetent skin. J Invest Dermatol 2010;130(8):2092–7.

29. Ferreira Cestari T, Hassun K, Sittart A, et al. A comparison of triple combination cream and hydroquinone 4% cream for the treatment of moderate to severe facial melasma. J Cosmet Dermatol 2007;6(1):36–9.

30. Monteiro RC, Kishore BN, Bhat RM, et al. A comparative study of the efficacy of 4% hydroquinone vs 0.75% kojic acid cream in the treatment of facial melasma. Indian J Dermatol 2013;58(2):157.

31. Deo KS, Dash KN, Sharma YK, et al. Kojic acid vis-a-vis its combinations with hydroquinone and betamethasone valerate in melasma: a randomized, single blind, comparative study of efficacy and safety. Indian J Dermatol 2013;58(4):281.

32. Bala HR, Lee S, Wong C, et al. Oral tranexamic acid for the treatment of melasma: a review. Dermatol Surg 2018;44(6):814–25.

33. Sadako N. Treatment of melasma with tranexamic acid. Clin Rep 1979;(13):3129–31.

34. Cho HH, Choi M, Cho S, et al. Role of oral tranexamic acid in melasma patients treated with IPL and low fluence QS Nd: YAG laser. J Dermatolog Treat 2013;24(4):292–6.

35. Li Y, Sun Q, He Z, et al. Treatment of melasma with oral administration of compound tranexamic acid: a preliminary clinical trial. J Eur Acad Dermatol Venereol 2014;28(3):393–4.

36. Shin JU, Park J, Oh SH, et al. Oral tranexamic acid enhances the efficacy of low-fluence 1064-nm quality-switched neodymium-doped yttrium aluminum garnet laser treatment for melasma in Koreans: a randomized, prospective trial. Dermatol Surg 2013;39(3 Pt 1):435–42.

37. Wu S, Shi H, Wu H, et al. Treatment of melasma with oral administration of tranexamic acid. Aesthetic Plast Surg 2012;36(4):964–70.

38. Na J, Choi S, Yang S, et al. Effect of tranexamic acid on melasma: a clinical trial with histological evaluation. J Eur Acad Dermatol Venereol 2013;27(8):1035–9.

39. Padhi T, Pradhan S. Oral tranexamic acid with fluocinolone-based triple combination cream versus fluocinolone-based triple combination cream alone in melasma: an open labeled randomized comparative trial. Indian J Dermatol 2015;60(5):520.

40. Lee HC, Thng TGS, Goh CL. Oral tranexamic acid (TA) in the treatment of melasma: a retrospective analysis. J Am Acad Dermatol 2016;75(2):385–92.

41. Del Rosario E, Florez-Pollack S, Zapata L Jr, et al. Randomized, placebo-controlled, double-blind study of oral tranexamic acid in the treatment of moderate-to-severe melasma. J Am Acad Dermatol 2018;78(2):363–9.

42. Maeda K, Tomita Y. Mechanism of the inhibitory effect of tranexamic acid on melanogenesis in cultured human melanocytes in the presence of keratinocyte-conditioned medium. J Health Sci 2007;53(4):389–96.

43. Taylor CR, Anderson RR. Ineffective treatment of refractory melasma and postinflammatory hyperpigmentation by Q-switched ruby laser. J Dermatol Surg Oncol 1994;20(9):592–7.

44. Tse Y, Levine VJ, McClain SA, et al. The removal of cutaneous pigmented lesions with the Q-switched ruby laser and the Q-switched neodymium: yttrium-aluminum-garnet laser. A comparative study. J Dermatol Surg Oncol 1994;20(12):795–800.

45. Hilton S, Heise H, Buhren BA, et al. Treatment of melasma in Caucasian patients using a novel 694-nm Q-switched ruby fractional laser. Eur J Med Res 2013;18:43.

46. Jang WS, Lee CK, Kim BJ, et al. Efficacy of 694-nm Q-switched ruby fractional laser treatment of melasma in female Korean patients. Dermatol Surg 2011;37(8):1133–40.

47. Fabi SG, Friedmann DP, Niwa Massaki AB, et al. A randomized, split-face clinical trial of low-fluence Q-switched neodymium-doped yttrium aluminum garnet (1,064 nm) laser versus low-fluence Q-switched alexandrite laser (755 nm) for the treatment of facial melasma. Lasers Surg Med 2014; 46(7):531–7.

48. Cho S, Kim J, Kim M. Melasma treatment in Korean women using a 1064-nm Q-switched Nd: YAG laser with low pulse energy. Clin Exp Dermatol 2009; 34(8):e847–50.

49. Brown AS, Hussain M, Goldberg DJ. Treatment of Melasma with low fluence, large spot size, 1064-nm Q-switched neodymium-doped yttrium aluminum garnet (Nd: YAG) laser for the treatment of melasma in Fitzpatrick skin types II–IV. J Cosmet Laser Ther 2011;13(6):280–2.

50. Wattanakrai P, Mornchan R, Eimpunth S. Low-fluence Q-switched neodymium-doped yttrium aluminum garnet (1,064 nm) laser for the treatment of facial melasma in Asians. Dermatol Surg 2010; 36(1):76–87.

51. Kasai K. Picosecond laser treatment for tattoos and benign cutaneous pigmented lesions (secondary publication). Laser Ther 2017;26(4):274–81.

52. Chalermchai T, Rummaneethorn P. Effects of a fractional picosecond 1,064 nm laser for the treatment of dermal and mixed type melasma. J Cosmet Laser Ther 2018;20(3):134–9.

53. Choi YJ, Nam JH, Kim JY, et al. Efficacy and safety of a novel picosecond laser using combination of 1 064 and 595 nm on patients with melasma: a prospective, randomized, multicenter, split-face, 2% hydroquinone cream-controlled clinical trial. Lasers Surg Med 2017;49(10):899–907.

54. Cho SB, Park SJ, Kim JS, et al. Treatment of postinflammatory hyperpigmentation using 1064-nm Q-switched Nd:YAG laser with low fluence: report of three cases. J Eur Acad Dermatol Venereol 2009; 23(10):1206–7.

55. Katz TM, Goldberg LH, Firoz BF, et al. Fractional photothermolysis for the treatment of postinflammatory hyperpigmentation. Dermatol Surg 2009;35(11): 1844–8.

56. Rokhsar CK, Ciocon DH. Fractional photothermolysis for the treatment of postinflammatory hyperpigmentation after carbon dioxide laser resurfacing. Dermatol Surg 2009;35(3):535–7.

57. Savory SA, Agim NG, Mao R, et al. Reliability assessment and validation of the postacne hyperpigmentation index (PAHPI), a new instrument to measure postinflammatory hyperpigmentation from acne vulgaris. J Am Acad Dermatol 2014;70(1): 108–14.

An Overview of Acne Therapy, Part 1
Topical therapy, Oral Antibiotics, Laser and Light Therapy, and Dietary Interventions

Justin W. Marson, BA[a], Hilary E. Baldwin, MD[b,c],*

KEYWORDS

- Acne • Treatment • Therapy • Antibiotic resistance • Adult female acne

KEY POINTS

- Research into the pathophysiology of acne over the last decade has defined the disorder to be principally one of innate immune dysfunction and inflammation.
- Efficacy of antibiotics in the treatment of acne, although indisputable, is largely related to their anti-inflammatory capabilities.
- Therapeutic regimens that limit the use of antibiotics have been proposed.
- Laser and light therapies are a potential non-antibiotic alternative for the treatment of acne. Modality choice, energy, and treatment frequency have not yet been fully elucidated.
- The role that diet plays in acne occurrence and severity has been inadequately studied, yet it remains one of the most pressing concerns for acne patients.

INTRODUCTION

Acne is a natural, but undesirable rite of passage during the teenage years sparing virtually no one.[1,2] Acne may also continue into adulthood, when the prevalence has been found to be statistically significantly higher in women at all age groups.[3] Although the prevalence decreases with time, a survey of 1013 participants found that it still affects 50% of women in their 20s, a third in their 30s, and a quarter in their 40s.[3] In all patients the physical and psychological scars can last a lifetime.[4] Therefore, because acne is such a common occurrence with immeasurable psychological trauma, we continue to search for the most efficacious and tolerable treatment regimens.

Therapeutic actives for acne have changed little in the last decade. Recognition that acne is an inflammatory, not infectious condition has led to a call for reduction in antibiotic use. This has culminated in a re-evaluation of highly efficacious combination topical therapy, improved vehicle technology, and a renaissance for spironolactone and isotretinoin (Justin W. Marson and Hilary E. Baldwin's article, "An Overview of Acne Therapy, Part 2: Hormonal Therapy and Isotretinoin," in this issue). Laser and light modalities, although not sufficiently studied for first-line use, show promise for the future.

It is important to realize that acute therapy, especially when acne is moderate-severe, may bear little resemblance to long-term maintenance therapy in the same patient. The goal of acute therapy is to make the patient significantly better as fast as possible; this generally requires multiple medications, frequently involving oral antibiotics.

Disclosure Statement: J.W. Marson: none. H.E. Baldwin: Speakers bureau for Galderma, Valeant, Sun, Mayne, Bayer. Investigator for Galderma, Valeant.
[a] Rutgers Robert Wood Johnson Medical School, 675 Hoes Lane West, Piscataway, NJ 08854, USA; [b] The Acne Treatment and Research Center, Morristown, NJ 07960, USA; [c] Rutgers Robert Wood Johnson Medical Center, New Brunswick, NJ 08901, USA
* Corresponding author. 310 Madison Avenue, Morristown, NJ 07960.
E-mail address: hbaldwin@acnetrc.com

Dermatol Clin 37 (2019) 183–193
https://doi.org/10.1016/j.det.2018.12.001
0733-8635/19/© 2018 Elsevier Inc. All rights reserved.

derm.theclinics.com

Once the patient has improved, having leapt the initial therapeutic hurdle, maintenance can often be accomplished with topical therapy alone, while it may have been too slow or insufficiently effective as initial therapy.

Products currently available for treating acne in the United States are summarized in **Box 1**. Each of these agents will be discussed individually recognizing that they will more often be used as part of a combination regimen. The role that diet plays in the initiation and continuation of acne is unclear but remains one of our patients' most frequently asked questions.

TOPICAL THERAPY
Antibacterials

Benzoyl peroxide
Benzoyl peroxide (BPO) is a potent antibacterial that has been shown not only to kill *Propionibacterium acnes* by the release of free radicals, but also to have mild comedolytic abilities.[5] It is available in a wide range of concentrations (2.5%–10%) and vehicles (cream, gel and foam leave-on, foam short-contact, and cleansers). Although effective as monotherapy, it is often used in conjunction with topical retinoids, which have been shown to augment BPO effectiveness.[6–8] Several fixed

---

Box 1
Available acne modalities

Topical therapies
  Antibacterial
    Benzoyl peroxide, clindamycin, erythromycin
  Retinoids
    Adapalene, tazarotene, tretinoin
  Others
    Dapsone, azelaic acid
Oral therapies
  Antibiotics
    Tetracyclines, macrolides, sulfamethoxazole, trimethoprim
  Hormonal therapy
    Oral contraceptives, spironolactone
  Isotretinoin
Procedural therapies
  Comedone extraction
  Chemical peels
  Laser
  Light

---

combination products using BPO 5% with erythromycin and BPO 2.5%, BPO 3.75%, and BPO 5% with clindamycin also show superiority over either agent alone.[9,10]

The most common side effect of BPO is concentration-dependent irritation, and vehicle development is of paramount importance in determining tolerability. Formulation considerations including micronization of the BPO and the inclusion of emollients can alter efficacy and tolerability, which precludes the assumption of equivalence by concentration alone.[11,12] Bleaching and staining of fabric is common, especially with leave-on formulations. Patients must be instructed to choose application time accordingly to avoid permanent damage of towels, sheets, and clothing.

Unlike other antibacterial agents used in acne, BPO has not been associated with the development of resistant *P acnes* strains.[12] The addition of leave-on BPO to regimens of topical and oral antibiotics has been shown to reduce emergence of resistant strains.[13] One branded BPO 6% cleanser was shown to not only reduce development of bacterial resistance, but to also reduce the population of already resistant *P acnes*.[14] Caution should be used when generalizing this finding to non-branded formulations in which substantivity of BPO has not been demonstrated.

Antibiotics

Topical antibiotics, namely erythromycin and clindamycin, are thought to work by 2 mechanisms: anti-microbial activity against *P acnes* and indirect anti-inflammatory effects.[15] Concomitant use of BPO (either as a leave-on or cleanser) is recommended to increase efficacy and decrease the development of resistant *P acnes* strains.[16,17] Use of topical clindamycin as monotherapy resulted in a dramatic increase in resistant strains as early as 2 months, whereas in combination with BPO 5% no such increase occurred.[13] Of the 2, clindamycin is the preferred agent as profound *P acnes* resistance to erythromycin has resulted in decreased clinically efficacy over time.[18] As mentioned above, several fixed combinations of clindamycin and BPO are available where efficacy of the combination was shown to be more efficacious than the monads.

Retinoids

Topical retinoids are vitamin A derivatives that have anti-inflammatory properties and reduce formation of the microcomedo by normalizing follicular hyperkeratinization. They have been shown to enhance the efficacy of other topical and oral regimens.[19] They are effective against existing comedonal and inflammatory lesions and preventative for future lesions.[16] Thus they are a part of acute and maintenance regimens.

Three active agents are currently available with more on the horizon: adapalene, tazarotene, and tretinoin. All have randomized, double-blinded, placebo-controlled trials demonstrating efficacy and safety.[20–23] Several formulations and concentrations of each active are available: tretinoin 0.025%–0.1% gel, cream, microsphere gel, and, most recently, lotion, adapalene 0.1% lotion and gel, 0.3% cream and tazarotene 0.05%–0.1% cream and gel, and 0.1% foam. Each retinoid binds to a different combination of retinoic acid receptors resulting in differences in efficacy and tolerability. Fixed combinations of tretinoin/clindamycin and adapalene/BPO are also available.

The most common side effect of topical retinoids is cutaneous irritation including stinging/burning, pruritus, erythema, and peeling. Irritation tends to peak at 1 to 2 weeks and decline thereafter despite continued use. Side effects can be mitigated by lowering the concentration, changing from gel to cream or lotion formulation, reducing the frequency of use and the concomitant use of moisturizers.[12,19] In general, increasing the concentration of the retinoid increases efficacy but may reduce tolerability.[20] Improved vehicle technology has gone a long way in reducing irritation with tretinoin, in which microsphere and micronized formulations have less irritation potential compared with standard tretinoin formulations.[24] Very recently tretinoin 0.05% lotion was introduced in which polymerized emulsion technology was used to improve efficacy and tolerability in patients as young as 9 years.[25] There are many head-to-head studies looking at the various actives, concentrations, and formulations in an effort to identify the more efficacious and more tolerable retinoid.[26–29] In general, the variability of these studies precludes direct comparisons.

All topical retinoids are associated with increased sun-sensitivity because of desquamation of the outer layers of the stratum corneum; as such, daily sunscreen use is recommended.[16] As a result of their similarity to oral retinoids, which are known teratogens, all topical retinoids share recommended limitations of use during pregnancy. This is primarily a theoretic concern as systemic absorption of all 3 topical actives is miniscule when used for acne and there is an absence of reports indicating retinoid-embryopathy when their use coincided with unintentional pregnancies.[30,31]

Tretinoin (but not microsphere formulation tretinoin, adapalene, or tazarotene) is not photo-stable and is best used in the evening. Tretinoin (but again not the others) is oxidized and inactivated by the presence of BPO, and sequential application is not recommended. Because co-application might be expected to improve compliance over twice-a-day application, use of the microsphere formulation of tretinoin or use of adapalene or tazarotene may be preferable when BPO is also being used.

Azelaic Acid

Azelaic acid 20% cream has numerous properties that may contribute to modest clinical efficacy in acne. It has been shown to be mildly comedolytic, antibacterial, and anti-inflammatory.[32] It also has a mild lightening effect on acne-induced hyperpigmentation.[33] Recently azelaic acid 15% foam, approved by the US Food and Drug Administration (FDA) for rosacea, was used in a small pilot open-label study in which it was found to be effective in reducing lesion count with good tolerability,[34] and was also shown to be helpful in the treatment of truncal acne.[35] Studies evaluating azelaic acid safety in animals and humans have shown it to be safe during pregnancy. As it is one of the only available agents in that patient population (along with metronidazole and clindamycin), that may be its most beneficial use.

Dapsone

Dapsone 7.5% gel is available as a once daily agent for acne. Its mechanism of action is not well understood; it is thought to function as an anti-inflammatory agent. Its efficacy has been evaluated in a large phase 3 trial.[36] It seems to be more efficacious against inflammatory than comedonal lesions and may be more effective in women than men and adolescents.[37–39] Dapsone gel is generally well-tolerated. Systemic absorption is minimal and the baseline testing of glucose-6-phosphate dehydrogenase was found to be unnecessary even in patients with known G6PD deficiency. Pharmacokinetic studies of the 7.5% every-day formulation indicate a reduction in systemic exposure compared with the 5.0% twice-a-day formulation.[40]

ORAL MEDICATIONS
Antibiotics

Oral antibiotics have been an integral component of acne therapy for decades. Efficacy has been demonstrated for the tetracycline class, trimethoprim/sulfamethoxazole (TMP/SMX), trimethoprim alone, the macrolides, amoxicillin, and cephalexin.[16,41] Owing to heterogeneity in study design and outcome measures, superior efficacy of one antibiotic over another cannot be determined and preference is often made based on side effect pro-files.[42] There is a similar dearth of data regarding optimal dosing, dosing frequency, and duration of treatment.

Antibiotics are highly effective for inflammatory acne because of their antibiotic activity and anti-inflammatory effects. This is particularly true of the tetracycline class of antibiotics whose numerous direct anti-inflammatory activities stem from the inhibition of matrix metalloproteinase ac-tivity, cytokine production, and chemotaxis.[43,44] As a result of their anti-inflammatory effects, but also their low cost, ease of administration, and excellent safety profile, the tetracyclines are considered first-line oral therapy for acne. The most recently developed minocycline preparation is minocycline hydrochloride extended-release tablets, which is used at 1 mg/kg once daily with similar efficacy to higher doses and markedly reduced vestibular side effects.[45]

Macrolides are most commonly used when tet-racyclines are not tolerated or contraindicated (eg, in pregnancy, patients younger than 8 years, and allergy).[16,46] Many authors suggest limiting the use of erythromycin because of worldwide resistance.[16,42] Azithromycin has been evaluated in many dosing regimens, often using pulse dosing of 3 doses/week to 4 days/month with good effi-cacy in open-label studies.[47–51] TMP/SMX, peni-cillins, and cephalosporins have limited data to support their use, which is largely limited to case reports.[52,53]

Although antibiotics are considered first-line therapy for moderate-severe acne, they are not (with the exception of extended-release minocy-cline), classically FDA-approved for this purpose. Technically, they are approved for adjunctive use only. However, this technicality is conveniently in keeping with guideline recommendations that oral antibiotics should always be used in combina-tion with BPO and/or a topical retinoid.[16,41,54,55] Numerous studies have shown that these combi-nations target varied pathophysiologic mecha-nisms,[19] work faster, achieve more complete clearance,[54,56–60] prolong remission rates,[58] and help to reduce the development of resistant *P acnes* strains.[19,46]

Side effects of the oral antibiotics used for acne differ with each agent. All tetracyclines are limited to patients ≥8 years of age owing to teratogenic effects and are associated with the rare occur-rence of idiopathic intracranial hypertension (pseudotumor cerebri).[60] The most common adverse effects of doxycycline are gastrointestinal distress and dose-dependent photosensi-tivity.[61,62] Gastrointestinal disturbances can be reduced by enteric coating, administration with a large glass of water and maintaining an erect posture for 30 to 60 minutes after dose administra-tion.[61–65] Common side effects seen with minocy-cline are vestibular in nature and are less common with the extended-release formulation.[45,64]

Minocycline is also uncommonly associated with pigment deposition in the skin and mucous mem-branes.[19,62,63] The risk of this side effect is related to cumulative exposure of the drug and increases with continued use, although the time of onset is un-predictable.[62] Pigmentation was not reported dur-ing the 2-year safety study with extended-release minocycline, perhaps because of the reduced exposure to drug with the 1 mg/kg dosing.[66]

Minocycline administration may be associated with the development of autoantibodies including anti-nuclear antibody. Although gener-ally asymptomatic, a lupus-like syndrome is rarely reported with complaints of arthralgias and malaise.[63] Spontaneous resolution occurs with discontinuation of the drug. Drug reaction with eosinophilia and systemic symptoms and other hypersensitivity reactions have also been rarely reported.[67–70]

Adverse effects of TMP/SMX include uncom-mon gastrointestinal disturbances and mild photo-sensitivity. Rare but potentially life-threatening drug eruptions, such as Stevens-Johnson syn-drome (SJS) and toxic epidermal necrolysis (TEN), and hematologic disorders, such as neutro-penia, aplastic anemia, and thrombocytopenia, have been reported.[71,72] SJS and TEN are rare, occurring in 4.5 patients/million users/week with a crude relative risk of 160 (aminopenicillins in the same study had a crude relative risk of 6.7). Both drug reactions are far more common in HIV-infected patients, and the highest risk seems to be within the first few weeks of use.[73] Periodic monitoring of the complete blood count is recom-mended when the drug is used long term.[16]

The macrolides, penicillins, and cephalosporins are associated with increased gastrointestinal dis-turbances. The penicillins, cephalosporins, and less commonly azithromycin, have been associ-ated with hypersensitivity reactions that can result in anaphylaxis.[16]

Antibiotic resistance

When discussing antibiotic resistance in the realm of oral antibiotics used for acne, 2 distinct issues arise. The first concerns *P acnes* resistance and begs the question: are patients with a high preva-lence of resistant strains unresponsive or less responsive to therapy? The second, and more important issue is the collateral damage on non-target bacteria and asks the question does anti-biotic use for acne cause disease?

P acnes resistance was first reported in 1979 and since then has been reported worldwide.[46,73] This is particularly true for erythromycin and clindamycin in which at least 50% of patients were found to be colonized with resistant P acnes.[74] With increasing prevalence of resistant strains, we as clinicians can anticipate a reduction or absence of response and an increase in relapse following antibiotic use.[24] Colonization with antibiotic-resistant strains has been shown to result in lessened response to erythromycin, tetracycline, minocycline, and oxytetracycline.[19,75,76] Younger clinicians may not recognize this deterioration as their expectations of response were formed in the era of resistance.

Antibiotic resistance is a major worldwide concern and the Centers for Disease Control (CDC) estimated that 23,000 deaths occurred in 2013 as a result of drug-resistant bacteria.[77] In acne, the use of topical and oral antibiotics was shown to result in a 3-fold increase of Streptococcus pyogenes colonization of the oropharynx compared with non-users.[78] Long-term use of topical and oral antibiotics in acne was associated with a statistically significant increase in upper respiratory infections,[79,80] multidrug-resistant glycemic index (GI) flora[81] and Staphylococcus aureus.[82] These data verify that concerns regarding prolonged use of antibiotics apply not only to P acnes and acne, but to the microbiome of other body locations where the dysbiosis of the commensal organisms can result in disease.

The CDC has issued a call to arms regarding antibiotic stewardship. To that end, as it applies to antibiotic use in acne, the consensus guidelines recommend use of antibiotics for a minimum of 6 to 8 weeks[19] limitation of use (if possible) to 3 months[16] or 6 months if necessary,[16,46] discontinuation if no response is seen after 12 weeks of therapy,[19] treatment of relapse with the same antibiotic that was previously effective,[19,61] consideration of anti-microbial dose doxycycline,[16] and avoiding monotherapy by always using oral antibiotics in combination with topical retinoids and or retinoid and BPO[16,19,42] (**Box 2**). The most recent guidelines of care from the American Academy of Dermatology, however, recognizes that there is a subset of patients who may require longer use of oral antibiotics when alternatives are contraindicated.[16]

DIETARY CONSIDERATIONS IN ACNE

The role of diet in the acne pathogenesis is controversial. Epidemiologic studies have found populations that follow a diet of low GI foods, dairy, and oils have vanishingly rare prevalence of acne.[83–87]

> **Box 2**
> **Consensus recommendations for oral antibiotics in acne**
>
> - Use for a minimum of 6 to 8 weeks
> - Limit use to 3 months, 6 months if necessary
> - Discontinuation if no response seen after 12 weeks of therapy
> - Use of sub-anti-microbial-dose doxycycline an initial or maintenance therapy
> - Repeat treatment, if necessary, should be with previously effective antibiotic
> - Consideration of anti-microbial dose doxycycline
> - Absence of monotherapy; always use in combination with topical retinoids or BPO/retinoids

---

However, with the adaptation of Western diet, these same populations began to develop acne.[84–87]

GI and Glycemic Load

Glycemic index is a ranking system of carbohydrate quality,[88] with higher values heaving a greater ability to increase blood glucose and serum insulin levels. Glycemic load (GL) considers the quality and quantity of the carbohydrate.[88] The most current framework suggest high GI/GL diets induce hyperinsulinemia and increase insulin-like growth factor 1 (IGF-1), thereby exacerbating keratinocyte proliferation and comedone formation.[89] In addition, hyperinsulinemia and elevated IGF-1 have been shown to augment androgen secretion thereby upregulating acetyl coenzyme A (CoA) carboxylase and stearoyl CoA desaturase activity leading to both hyperseborrhea and dysseborrhea (respectively), which, via P acnes, drives inflammation.[89]

A literature review assessed metformin as an adjunct for acne therapy (either topicals or topicals and oral antibiotics) and found, in 3 trials, some evidence that individuals with acne who received metformin had greater reduction in total lesion counts and inflammatory lesions from baseline compared with their control counterparts with minimal side effects (eg, diarrhea and flatulence).[90]

Randomized controlled trials have shown that low GI/GL diets can mitigate acne severity, increase insulin sensitivity and IGF binding proteins 1 and 3, and increase proportion of saturated fatty acids to monounsaturated fatty acids in sebum compared with controls on a classic Western diet; however, many trials have been unable to separate the effects of diet from weight loss.[91–95]

Dairy

Several retrospective and prospective survey-based studies have primarily implicated skim milk in the pathogenesis of acne.[96,97] Adebamowo and colleagues[96,97] hypothesized that processing whole-fat milk into skim milk increases the bioavailability of compounds, such as casein and whey, that instigate acne.

Interestingly, a 2017 longitudinal study found contrary correlations between high intake (2 or more servings daily) of full-fat dairy products with acne and high intake of total dairy and acne among women.[98] A 2018 meta-analysis of 14 studies found a linear dose-response for total dairy, skim milk, and whole-fat milk, wherein each additional serving increased the risk of acne by 83%, 26%, and 13%, respectively; they also found a non-linear dose-response relationship between total dairy, total milk, low-fat milk, skim milk, and acne.[99]

Though not well understood, it is thought that casein and whey within dairy may independently elevate IGF-1 and promote comedogenesis and sebaceous lipogenesis by stimulating gonadal androgenesis and inhibiting of hepatic-derived sex-hormone binding globulins.[99] This is supported by multiple case reports and a case series documenting new onset or recalcitrant nodular cystic acne coinciding with the use of whey protein supplements, an assortment of globular dairy proteins popular among bodybuilders and weight-lifters.[100–102] The largest of the current studies followed 30 individuals using predominately whey protein-based supplements for 2 months and found significant increases in inflammatory papules (15.8 vs 1.87, $P<.0005$), pustules (14 vs 0.3, $P<.0005$), and non-inflammatory lesions (19.7 vs 11.8, $P = .002$), compared with baseline.[102]

Other Dietary Issues

There are also several randomized-controlled trials that have investigated the use of foods or food supplements as possible adjuncts in acne therapy. There is some evidence that low levels of omega-3 poly-unsaturated fatty acids (PUFAs) contribute to an inflammatory state in individuals with acne.[103–105] Furthermore, at least 1 double-blind randomized-control trial showed improvement of inflammatory and non-inflammatory lesions with 10 weeks of oral supplementation with either omega-3 PUFA or an anti-inflammatory omega-6 gamma-linolenic acid.[105]

LASER- AND LIGHT-BASED THERAPIES

Laser- and light-based therapies (LBTs) are novel, non-antibiotic therapies new to the acne regimen.

Their currently understood therapeutic mechanism of action includes: (1) light, (2) photosensitive adjunct, and (3) reactive oxidative species (ROS). Endogenous (porphyrins found in *P acnes*) or exogenously applied photosensitive adjuncts (photodynamic therapy [PDT]) are excited by light and create ROS targeted either at *P acnes* or the sebaceous gland, reducing inflammation and sebum production.[106]

A 2018 Cochrane systematic review by Barbaric and colleagues[106] compiled current data about the use of different modalities of light therapy and found mixed results for their use in acne. In assessing PDT, Barbaric and colleagues found no current evidence to support aminolevulinic acid (ALA)-PDT with blue light as participants' global assessment of improvement showed no benefit over blue light alone. They found weak evidence for the use of 15% –10% ALA-PDT with non-blue light (ie, red light and intense pulsed light [IPL]) given findings that 15% ALA with red light had similar efficacy as 20% ALA with red light with decreased adverse effects (eg, blistering), and that 10% ALA with IPL was superior to IPL alone in reducing inflammatory and non-inflammatory lesions. They also found that methyl aminolevulinate PDT with red light was no better at reducing either inflammatory or non-inflammatory lesions than placebo cream and red light.[106] Barbaric and colleagues[106] also included other forms of LBTs in their analysis but were hampered by the heterogeneous nature of the studies and paucity of raw data available. Although they found weak evidence for the use of blue-red light and similar efficacy of blue light to BPO, they could not find currently clinically significant evidence for the use of infrared light, yellow light, or gold microparticles.

As part of a larger review of non-pharmacological therapies for acne, de Vries and colleagues[107] also reported on the ability of different LBTs to reduce acne lesions compared with either a control or baseline.[107] They found moderate evidence for the use of single-pass IPL in reduction of both inflammatory and non-inflammatory acne lesions compared with double pass and the use of diode laser in reduction of inflammatory lesions compared with no treatment. They also included several studies that compared light therapies with more conventional therapies (blue light vs 1% clindamycin, blue light vs cumulative 54 mg/kg isotretinoin, IPL vs BPO, PDL vs 5% BPO gel and 0.1% tretinoin cream vs tetrachloroacetic acid). In all light-conventional head-to-head studies, there were no significant differences between treatment groups, suggesting non-inferiority of LBTs.

Most of the reported findings compared different forms of LBTs against each other or showed improvement over no therapy. Despite the quality of evidence being hampered by the methodology of the studies, many of the LBTs analyzed by de Vries and colleagues reported a "significant reduction" in acne lesions. As both the de Vries and Barbaric groups have justly noted, more stringently designed studies are needed to determine the role of LBTs, as adjunct or even monotherapy.

SUMMARY

Pharmacologic acne therapies have changed little in the past decade. The introduction of topical dapsone, improvement in vehicle technology, and progress in oral delivery systems account for the biggest changes. These improvements should not be minimized as improved topical and oral delivery have been shown to improve efficacy and tolerability. Although the efficacy and place of laser and light technology has not yet been clearly defined within the anti-acne arsenal, great strides have been made toward becoming first-line therapy. Additional data have been shed on the contribution of diet in acne occurrence and severity. The greatest changes, however, have been in recognizing the imminent threat of antibiotic resistance not only as a challenge in treating acne, but a global health crisis. Our increased understanding of antibiotic resistance has resulted in a better definition of acute and maintenance acne therapy. No longer are antibiotics considered a long-term treatment option. This has resulted in a renewed interest in existing alternative therapies. A renaissance for acne therapy is upon us, revitalizing the use of BPO and its ability to reduce the development of resistant bacteria and re-invoking the utility of topical retinoids for maintenance therapy.

REFERENCES

1. Tan J, Bhake K. A global perspective on the epidemiology of acne. Br J Dermatol 2015;172(Suppl 1): 3–12.
2. Bhake K, Williams H. Epidemiology acne vulgaris. Br J Dermatol 2013;168(3):474–85.
3. Collier C, Harper J, Cafardi J, et al. The prevalence of acne in adults 20 years and older. J Am Acad Dermatol 2008;58(5):874.
4. Layton A, Seukeran D, Cunliffe W. Scarred for life? Dermatology 1997;195(Suppl 1):15–21.
5. Fulton J, Farzad-Bakshandeh A, Bradley S. Studies on the mechanism of action of topical benzoyl peroxide and vitamin A acid in acne vulgaris. J Cutan Pathol 1974;1:191–200.
6. Shalita R, Rafal E, Anderson D, et al. Compared efficacy and safety of tretinoin 0.1% microsphere gel alone and in combination with benzoyl peroxide 6% cleanser for the treatment of acne vulgaris. Cutis 2003;72:167–72.
7. Tanghetti E, Abramivits W, Solomon B, et al. Tazarotene versus tazarotene plus clindamycin/benzoyl peroxide in the treatment of acne vulgaris: a multicenter, double-blind, randomized, parallel-group trial. J Drugs Dermatol 2006; 5(3):256–61.
8. Del Rosso J. Study results of benzoyl peroxide 5%/clindamycin 1% gel, adapalene 0.1% gel, and use in combination for acne vulgaris. J Drugs Dermatol 2007;6:616–22.
9. Seidler E, Kimball A. Meta-analysis of randomized controlled trials using 5% benzoyl peroxide and clindamycin versus 2.5% benzoyl peroxide and clindamycin in acne. J Am Acad Dermatol 2011; 65(4):3117–9.
10. Pariser D, Rich P, Cook-Bolden F, et al. An aqueous gel fixed combination of clindamycin phosphate 1.2% and benzoyl peroxide 3.75% for the once-daily treatment of moderate to severe acne. J Drugs Dermatol 2014;13(9):1083–9.
11. Tanghetti E, Popp K. A current review of topical benzoyl peroxide: new perspectives on formulation and utilization. Dermatol Clin 2009;27: 17–24.
12. Del Rosso J, Baldwin H, Keri J. Current approach to acne management: a community-based analysis. Cutis 2009;83(suppl 6):5–21.
13. Cunliffe W, Holland K, Bojar R, et al. A randomized, double-blind comparison of a clindamycin phosphate/benzoyl peroxide gel formulation and a matching clindamycin gel with respect to microbiologic activity and clinical efficacy in the topical treatment of acne vulgaris. Clin Ther 2002;24: 1117–33.
14. Leyden J. Antibiotic resistant *Propionibacterium acnes* suppressed by a benzoyl peroxide cleanser 6%. Cutis 2008;82(6):417–21.
15. Mills O, Thornsberry C, Cardin C, et al. Bacterial resistance and therapeutic outcome following three months of topical acne therapy with 2% erythromycin gel versus its vehicle. Acta Derm Venereol 2002;82:260–5.
16. Zaenglein A, Pathy A, Schlosser B, et al. Guidelines of care for the treatment of acne vulgaris. J Am Acad Dermatol 2016;74(5):945–73.
17. Leyden J, Del Rosso J, Webster G. Clinical considerations in the treatment of acne vulgaris and other inflammatory skin disorders: focus on antibiotic resistance. Cutis 2007;79(suppl 6):9–25.
18. Simonart T, Dramaix M. Treatment of acne with topical antibiotics: lessons from clinical studies. Br J Dermatol 2005;153:395–403.

19. Gollnick H, Cunliffe W, Berson D, et al. Global alliance to improve outcomes in acne. Management of acne: a report from a global alliance to improve outcomes in acne. J Am Acad Dermatol 2003; 49(suppl 1):S1–37.

20. Krishman G. Comparison of two concentrations of tretinoin solution in the topical treatment of acne vulgaris. Practitioner 1976;216:106–9.

21. Shalita A, Chalker D, Griffith R, et al. Tazarotene gel is safe and effective in the treatment of acne vulgaris: a multicenter, double-blind, vehicle-controlled study. Cutis 1999;63:349–54.

22. Lucky A, Cullen S, Funicella T, et al. Double-blind, vehicle-controlled, multicenter comparison of two 0.025% tretinoin creams in patients with acne vulgaris. J Am Acad Dermatol 1998;38: S24–30.

23. Pedace F, Stoughton R. Topical retinoic acid in acne vulgaris. Br J Dermatol 1971;84:465–9.

24. Del Rosso J. The role of the vehicle in combination acne therapy. Cutis 2005;76(suppl 2):15–8.

25. Tyring S, Kircik L, Pariser D, et al. Novel tretinoin 0.05% lotion for the once daily treatment of moderate-to-severe acne vulgaris: assessment of efficacy and safety in patients aged 9 and older. J Drugs Dermatol 2018;17(1):602–9.

26. Shalita A, Weiss J, Chalker D, et al. A comparison of the efficacy and safety of adapalene gel 0.1% and tretinoin gel 0.025% in the treatment of acne vulgaris: a multicenter trial. J Am Acad Dermatol 1996;34:482–5.

27. Dunlap F, Mills O, Tuley M, et al. Adapalene 0.1% gel for the treatment of acne vulgaris: its superiority compared to tretinoin 0.025% cream in skin tolerance and patient preference. Br J Dermatol 1998; 139:17–22.

28. Kakita L. Tazarotene versus tretinoin or adapalene in the treatment of acne vulgaris. J Am Acad Dermatol 2000;43:551–4.

29. Webster G, Berson D, Stein L, et al. Efficacy and tolerability of once-daily tazarotene 0.1% gel versus once-daily tretinoin 0.025% gel in the treatment of facial acne vulgaris: a randomized trial. Cutis 2001;67:4–9.

30. Panchaud A, Csajka C, Merlob P, et al. Pregnancy outcome following exposure to topical retinoids: a multicenter prospective study. J Clin Pharmacol 2012;52(12):1844–51.

31. Loureiro K, Kao K, Jones K. Minor malformations characteristic of the retinoid acid embryopathy and other birth outcomes in children of women exposed to topical tretinoin during early pregnancy. Am J Med Genet A 2005;136(2): 117–21.

32. Shulte B, Wu W, Rosen T. Azelaic acid: evidence-based update on mechanism of acne and clinical applications. J Drugs Dermatol 2015;14(9):964–8.

33. Kircik L. Efficacy and safety of azelaic acid (AzA) gel 15% in the treatment of post-inflammatory hyperpigmentation and acne: a 16 week, baseline-controlled study. J Drugs Dermatol 2011;10: 586–90.

34. Hashim P, Chen T, Harper J, et al. The efficacy and safety of azelaic acid 15% foam in the treatment of facial acne vulgaris. J Drugs Dermatol 2018;17(6): 641–5.

35. Hoffman L, Del Rosso J, Kircik L. The efficacy and safety of azelaic acid 15% foam in the treatment of truncal acne vulgaris. J Drugs Dermatol 2017; 16(6):534–8.

36. Stein Gold L, Jarratt M, Bucko A, et al. Efficacy and safety of once daily dapsone gel 7.5% for treatment of adolescents and adults with acne vulgaris: first of 2 identically designed, large, multicenter, randomized, vehicle-controlled trials. J Drugs Dermatol 2016;15(5):553–61.

37. Draelos Z, Carter E, Maloney J, et al. Two randomized studies demonstrate the efficacy and safety of dapsone gel, 5% for the treatment of acne vulgaris. J Am Acad Dermatol 2007;56: 439.e1-e10.

38. Tanghetti E, Harper J, Oefelein M. The efficacy and tolerability of dapsone 5% gel in female vs. male patients with facial acne vulgaris: gender as a clinically relevant outcome variable. J Drugs Dermatol 2012;11:1417–21.

39. Del Rosso J, Kircik L, Gallagher C. Comparative efficacy and tolerability of dapsone 5% gel in adult versus adolescent females with acne vulgaris. J Clin Aesthet Dermatol 2015;8:31–7.

40. Jarratt M, Jones T, Chang-Liu J, et al. Safety and pharmacokinetics of once-daily dapsone gel, 7.5% in patients with moderate acne vulgaris. J Drugs Dermatol 2016;15(10):1250–9.

41. Bienenfeld A, Nagler A, Orlow S. Oral antibiotic therapy for acne vulgaris: an evidence-based review. Am J Clin Dermatol 2017;18(4):469–90.

42. Eichenfield L, Krakowski A, Piggott C, et al. Evidence-based recommendations for the diagnosis and treatment of pediatric acne. Pediatrics 2013; 131(Suppl):S1–50.

43. Perret L, Tait C. Non-antibiotic properties of tetracycline and their clinical applications in dermatology. Australas J Dermatol 2014;55(2): 111–8.

44. Henehan M, Montuno M, DeBenedetto A. Doxycycline as an anti-inflammatory agent: updates in dermatology. J Eur Acad Dermatol Venereol 2017; 31(11):1800–8.

45. Fleischer A, Dinehart S, Stough D, et al. Solodyn Phase 2 and Phase 3 Study Group. Safety and efficacy of a new extended-release formulation of minocycline. Cutis 2006;78(suppl4): 21–31.

46. Dreno B, Bettoli V, Ochsendorf F, et al. European recommendations on the use of oral antibiotics for acne. Eur J Dermatol 2004;14(6):391–9.

47. Maleszka R, Turek-Urasinska K, Oremus M, et al. Pulsed azithromycin treatment is as effective and safe as 2-week-longer daily doxycycline treatment of acne vulgaris: a randomized, double-blind, non-inferiority study. Skinmed 2011;9:86–94.

48. Antonio J, Pegas J, Cestari T, et al. Azithromycin pulses in the treatment of inflammatory and pustular acne: efficacy, tolerability and safety. J Dermatolog Treat 2008;19:210–5.

49. Innocenzi D, Skroza N, Rugiero A, et al. Moderate acne vulgaris: efficacy, tolerance and compliance of oral azithromycin thrice weekly for. Acta Dermatovenerol Croat 2008;16:13–8.

50. Bardazzi F, Savoia F, Parente G, et al. Azithromycin: a new therapeutical strategy for acne in adolescents. Dermatol Online J 2007;13:4.

51. Basta-Juzbasic A, Lipozencic J, Oremovic L, et al. A dose-finding study of azithromycin in the treatment of acne vulgaris. Acta Dermatovenerol Croat 2007;15:141–7.

52. Jen I. A comparison of low dosage trimethoprim/sulfamethoxazole with oxytetracycline in acne vulgaris. Cutis 1980;26:106–8.

53. Fenner J, Wiss K, Levin N. Oral cephalexin for acne vulgaris: clinical experience with 93 patients. Pediatr Dermatol 2008;25:179–83.

54. Gold L, Cruz A, Eichenfield L, et al. Effective and safe combination therapy for severe acne vulgaris: a randomized, vehicle-controlled, double-blind study of adapalene 0.1%-benzoyl peroxide 2.5% fixed-dose combination gel with doxycycline hyclate 100 mg. Cutis 2010;85:94–104.

55. Zaenglein A, Shamban A, Webster G, et al. A phase IV, open-label study evaluating the use of triple-combination therapy with minocycline HCl extended-release tablets, a topical antibiotic-retinoid preparation and benzoyl peroxide in patients with moderate to severe acne vulgaris. J Drugs Dermatol 2013;12:619–25.

56. Thiboutot D, Shalita A, Yamauchi P, et al. Combination therapy with adapalene gel 0.1% and doxycycline for severe acne vulgaris: a multicenter, investigator blind, randomized, controlled study. Skinmed 2005;4(3):138–46.

57. Cunliffe W, Meynadier J, Alirezai M, et al. Is combined oral and topical therapy better than oral therapy alone in patients with moderate to moderately severe acne vulgaris? A comparison of the efficacy and safety of lymecycline plus adapalene gel 0.1% versus lymecycline plus gel vehicle. J Am Acad Dermatol 2003;49(3 Suppl):S218–26.

58. Tan J, Stein Gold L, Schlessinger J, et al. Short-term combination therapy and long-term relapse prevention in the treatment of severe acne vulgaris. J Drugs Dermatol 2012;11(2):174–80.

59. Dreno B, Kaufmann R, Talarico S, et al. Combination therapy with adapalene-benzoyl peroxide and oral lymecycline in the treatment of moderate to severe acne vulgaris; a multicentre, randomized, double-blind controlled study. Br J Dermatol 2011;165(2):383–90.

60. Del Rosso J. Systemic therapy for rosacea: focus on oral antibiotic therapy and safety. Cutis 2000;66(Suppl 4):7–13.

61. Del Rosso J, Kim G. Optimizing use of oral antibiotics in acne vulgaris. Dermatol Clin 2009;27:33–42.

62. Leyden J, Bruce S, Lee C, et al. A randomized, phase 2, dose-ranging study in the treatment of moderate to severe inflammatory facial acne vulgaris with doxycycline calcium. J Drugs Dermatol 2013;12:653–68.

63. Kircik L. Doxycycline and minocycline for the management of acne: a review of efficacy and safety with emphasis on clinical implications. J Drugs Dermatol 2010;9(11):1407–11.

64. Jarvinen A, Nykanen S, Paasiniemi L, et al. Enteric coating reduces upper gastrointestinal adverse reactions to doxycycline. Clin Drug Investig 1995;10(6):323–7.

65. Berger R. A double-blind, multiple-dose, placebo-controlled, cross-over study to compare the incidence of gastrointestinal complaints in healthy subjects given Doryx R and Vibramycin R. J Clin Pharmacol 1988;28:367–70.

66. Data on file. Clinical study report for MP-0104-07. Scottsdale (AZ): Medicis Pharmaceutical Corporation; 2007.

67. Kermani T, Ham E, Camilleri M, et al. Polyarteritis nodosa-like vasculitis in association with minocycline use: a single-center case series. Semin Arthritis Rheum 2012;42:213–21.

68. Shaughnessy K, Bouchard S, Mohn M, et al. Minocycline-induced drug reaction with eosinophilia and systemic symptoms (DRESS) syndrome with persistent myocarditis. J Am Acad Dermatol 2010;62:15–318.

69. Smith K, Leyden J. Safety of doxycycline and minocycline: a systematic review. Clin Ther 2005;27:1329–42.

70. Weinstein M, Laxer R, Debosz J, et al. Doxycycline-induced cutaneous inflammation with systemic symptoms in a patient with acne vulgaris. J Cutan Med Surg 2013;17:283–6.

71. Roujeau J, Kelly J, Naldi L. Medication use and the risk of Stevens-Johnson syndrome or toxic epidermal necrolysis. N Engl J Med 1995;333:1600–7.

72. Firoz B, Henning J, Zarzabal L, et al. Toxic epidermal necrolysis: five years of treatment experience from a burn unit. J Am Acad Dermatol 2012; 67:630–5.

73. Coopman S, Stern R. Cutaneous drug reactions in human immunodeficiency virus infection. Arch Dermatol 1991;127(5):714–7.

74. Ross J, Snelling A, Carnegie E, et al. Antibiotic-resistant acne: lessons from Europe. Br J Dermatol 2003;148(3):467–78.

75. Eady E, Cove J, Holland K, et al. Erythromycin resistant propionibacteria in antibiotic treated acne patients: association with therapeutic failure. Br J Dermatol 1989;121(1):51–7.

76. Leyden J, McGinley K, Cavalieri S, et al. Propionibacterium acnes resistance to antibiotics in acne patients. J Am Acad Dermatol 1983;8(1): 4105.

77. Antibiotic resistance threats in the United States. Centers for Disease control and Prevention; 2013. Available at: www.cdc.gov/drugresistance/pdf/ar-threats-2013-508.pdf.

78. Levy R, Huang E, Roling D, et al. Effect of antibiotics on the oropharyngeal flora in patients with acne. Arch Dermatol 2003;139(4):467–71.

79. Margolis D, Bowe W, Hoffstad O, et al. Antibiotic treatment of acne may be associated with upper respiratory tract infections. Arch Dermatol 2005; 141(9):1132–6.

80. Margolis D, Fanelli M, Kuperman E, et al. Association of pharyngitis with oral antibiotic use for the treatment of acne: a cross-sectional and prospective cohort study. Arch Dermatol 2012;148(3): 326–32.

81. Adams S, Cunliffe W, Cooke E. Long-term antibiotic therapy for acne vulgaris effects on the bowel flora of patients and their relatives. J Invest Dermatol 1985;85(1):35–7.

82. Patel M, Bowe W, Heughebaert C, et al. The development of antimicrobial resistance due to the antibiotic treatment of acne vulgaris: a review. J Drugs Dermatol 2010;9(6):655–64.

83. Cordain L, Lindeberg S, Hurtado M, et al. Acne vulgaris: a disease of Western civilization. Arch Dermatol 2002;138:1584–90.

84. Schaefer O. When the Eskimo comes to town. Nutr Today 1971;6:8–16.

85. Bendiner E. Disastrous trade-off: Eskimo health for white 'Civilization'. Hosp Pract 1974; 9:56–89.

86. Shen Y, Wang T, Zhou C, et al. Necropsies on Okinawans: anatomic and pathologic observations. Arch Pathol 1946;42:359–80.

87. Lynn DD, Umari T, Dunnick CA, et al. The epidemiology of acne vulgaris in late adolescence. Adolesc Health Med Ther 2016;7: 13–25.

88. Foster-Powell K, Holt S, Brand-Miller J. International table of glycemic index and glycemic load values: 2002. Am J Clin Nutr 2002;76:5–56.

89. Melnik B. Acne vulgaris: the metabolic syndrome of the pilosebaceous follicle. Clin Dermatol 2018;36: 29–40.

90. Lee J, Smith A. Metformin as an adjunct therapy for the treatment of moderate to severe acne vulgaris. Dermatol Online J 2017;23 [pii:13030/qt53m2q13s].

91. Burris J, Rietkerk W, Shikany J, et al. Differences in dietary glycemic load and hormones in New York City adults with no and moderate/severe acne. J Acad Nutr Diet 2017;117: 1375–83.

92. Kucharska A, Szmurlo A, Sinska B. Significance of diet in treated and untreated acne vulgaris. Postepy Dermatol Alergol 2016;33:81–6.

93. Smith R, Mann N, Braue A, et al. The effect of a high-protein, low glycemic-load diet versus a conventional, high glycemic-load diet on biochemical parameters associated with acne vulgaris: a randomized, investigator-masked, controlled trial. J Am Acad Dermatol 2007;57: 247–56.

94. Kwon H, Yoon J, Hong J, et al. Clinical and histological effect of a low glycaemic load diet in treatment of acne vulgaris in Korean patients: a randomized, controlled trial. Acta Derm Venereol 2012;92:241–6.

95. Smith R, Braue A, Varigos G, et al. The effect of a low glycemic load diet on acne vulgaris and the fatty acid composition of skin surface triglycerides. J Dermatol Sci 2008;50:41–52.

96. Adebamowo C, Spiegelman D, Danby F, et al. High school dietary dairy intake and teenage acne. J Am Acad Dermatol 2005;52:207–14.

97. Adebamowo C, Spiegelman D, Berkey C, et al. Milk consumption and acne in teenaged boys. J Am Acad Dermatol 2008;58:787–93.

98. Ulvestad M, Bjertness E, Dalgard F. Acne and dairy products in adolescence: results from a Norwegian longitudinal study. J Eur Acad Dermatol Venereol 2017;31:530–5.

99. Aghasi M, Golzarand M, Shab-Bidar S, et al. Dairy intake and acne development: a meta-analysis of observational studies. Clin Nutr 2018. https://doi.org/10.1016/j.clnu.2018.04.015.

100. Silverberg N. Whey protein precipitating moderate to severe acne flares in 5 teenaged athletes. Cutis 2012;90:70–2.

101. Simonart T. Acne and whey protein supplementation among bodybuilders. Dermatology 2012;225: 256–8.

102. Pontes Tde C, Fernandes Filho G, Trindade Ade S, et al. Incidence of acne vulgaris in young adult users of protein-calorie supplements in the city of

Joao Pessoa–PB. An Bras Dermatol 2013;88: 907–12.

103. Rubin M, Kim K, Logan A. Acne vulgaris, mental health and omega-3 fatty acids: a report of cases. Lipids Health Dis 2008;7:36.

104. Aslan I. Decreased eicosapentaenoic acid levels in acne vulgaris reveals the presence of a proinflammatory state. Prostaglandins Other Lipid Mediat 2017;128-129:1–7.

105. Jung J, Kwon HH, Hong JS, et al. Effect of dietary supplementation with omega-3 fatty acid and gamma-linolenic acid on acne vulgaris: a randomised, double-blind, controlled trial. Acta Derm Venereol 2014;94(5):521–5.

106. Barbaric J, Abbott R, Posadzki P, et al. Light therapies for acne: abridged Cochrane systematic review including GRADE assessments. Br J Dermatol 2018;178(1):61–75.

107. de Vries F, Meulendijks AM, Driessen RJB, et al. The efficacy and safety of non-pharmacological therapies for the treatment of acne vulgaris: a systematic review and best-evidence synthesis. J Eur Acad Dermatol Venereol 2018;32(7): 1195–203.

An Overview of Acne Therapy, Part 2
Hormonal Therapy and Isotretinoin

Justin W. Marson, BA[a], Hilary E. Baldwin, MD[b,c],*

KEYWORDS

- Acne • Treatment • Therapy • Antibiotic resistance • Adult female acne

KEY POINTS

- Acne as an inflammatory condition is driven by multiple factors, including hormonal dysregulation.
- Spironolactone is an efficacious treatment for women with acne, and is safe for long-term use and precludes the use of antibiotics.
- Quality clinical trials have demonstrated a larger safety margin for isotretinoin than previously thought.

INTRODUCTION

Therapeutic actives for acne have changed little in the last decade. However, a major paradigm shift has occurred with the recognition that acne is an inflammatory, not infectious condition, which has led to a call for reduction in antibiotic use against the background of increasing reports of worldwide antibiotic resistance. Over the past 10 years there has been a re-evaluation of highly efficacious combination topical therapy (discussed in Part 1), and a renaissance for spironolactone and isotretinoin (**Box 1**).

Acne as an inflammatory condition is driven by multiple factors, including hormonal dysregulation. Recent studies have primed hormonal therapies for a resurgence demonstrating that not only are they efficacious, but safe with little need for continual monitoring. Isotretinoin safety has been evaluated in numerous studies that cumulatively suggest that although there are very real potential adverse events including teratogenicity and mimicry of hypervitaminosis A, the drug is much safer than an Internet search purports it to be. The potential adverse effects must be weighed against the fact that only isotretinoin addresses all facets of acne pathogenesis and only isotretinoin possesses the potential to cure rather than control acne.

HORMONAL THERAPY

For women with acne, hormonal therapy provides an excellent treatment option. This group of agents targets the important role of androgens in the pathogenesis of acne. Hormonal therapy was recommended by previous guidelines as an alternative to systemic antibiotics and/or isotretinoin for the treatment of moderate to severe acne in women. However, in the last 5 to 10 years it has achieved first-line status.[1–5] Common options in the United States include combined oral contraceptives (COCs) and spironolactone. Both agents inhibit binding of testosterone to androgen receptors, and conversion of testosterone to dihydrotestosterone; they also increase sex hormone-binding globulin, which reduces free testosterone in the blood.[6,7] In addition, local overproduction

Disclosure Statement: J.W. Marson: none. Dr H.E. Baldwin: Speakers bureau for Galderma, Valeant, Sun, Mayne, Bayer. Investigator for Galderma, Valeant.

[a] Rutgers Robert Wood Johnson Medical School, 675 Hoes Lane West, Piscataway, NJ 08854, USA; [b] The Acne Treatment and Research Center, Morristown, NJ 07960, USA; [c] Rutgers Robert Wood Johnson Medical Center, New Brunswick, NJ 08901, USA

* Corresponding author. 310 Madison Avenue, Morristown, NJ 07960.

E-mail address: hbaldwin@acnetrc.com

Dermatol Clin 37 (2019) 195–203
https://doi.org/10.1016/j.det.2018.12.002
0733-8635/19/© 2018 Elsevier Inc. All rights reserved.

Box 1
Available acne modalities

Topical therapies

Antibacterial

Benzoyl peroxide, clindamycin, erythromycin

Retinoids

Adapalene, tazarotene, tretinoin

Others

Dapsone, azelaic acid

Oral therapies

Antibiotics

Tetracyclines, macrolides, sulfamethoxazole, trimethoprim

Hormonal therapy

Oral contraceptives, spironolactone

Isotretinoin

Procedural therapies

Comedone extraction

Chemical peels

of androgens or androgen receptor hypersensitivity may play a role,[8] which may explain the finding that hormonal therapy is effective even in patients with normal serum androgens. This population constitutes the majority of women with acne who individually have levels of circulating androgens within normal limits. It should be noted that in a study comparing androgen levels in women with and without acne, the mean levels of androgens were higher in the group with acne.[9]

Combination Oral Contraceptives

All COCs contain ethinyl estradiol (EE) in varied dosages and a progestational moiety. Since their development in 1960, EE levels have gradually decreased with an overall improvement in safety profile. At the same time the progestins have undergone 4 iterations. First-, second-, and third-generation progestins are developed from testosterone and as such, if used as monotherapy, have androgenic potential. Fourth-generation progestins, including drospirenone are not developed from testosterone. Despite the contribution of the various progestins, once combined with EE the net effect of all COCs is antiandrogenic.[10] Therefore all COCs are theoretically useful in the treatment of acne, although only 4 have gone through the rigorous Food and Drug Administration (FDA) testing necessary to acquire the indication for

acne. The 4 FDA-approved COCs in the United States have as their progestin moiety norgestimate (Ortho Tri-Cyclen), norethindrone acetate (Estrostep Fe), drospirenone (Yaz), and drospirenone with the addition of levomefolic acid (Beyaz) (**Table 1**).

Efficacy of the COCs has been demonstrated in numerous randomized and controlled clinical trials.[11–17] Statistically significant improvements have been shown in treatment success alongside reduction in both inflammatory and noninflammatory lesions and patient self-assessments. Owing to variations in study design, superiority of one agent over another in the treatment of acne is unclear.[1,9] Onset of action is generally slow, with clinical improvement often not appreciated until 3 to 6 months.[11,14–16] Combination of COCs with other medications at initiation of therapy is generally warranted.

The side effects of COCs have been evaluated in millions of women.[18] Overall there are similar mortality rates seen between users and nonusers, but side effects are frequent and differ according to EE dose and progestin type.[19] Common side effects seen with COC use include weight gain, breast tenderness, breakthrough bleeding, and moodiness, all of which are seen less frequently with the newer-generation COCs. More serious side effects are fortunately uncommon and include venous thromboembolism (VTE), stroke, and myocardial infarction. Again the risk of these side effects has been reduced with the low-dose COCs, which include all of the COCs approved by the FDA for acne.[20,21] COC use is contraindicated in women with poorly controlled hypertension, migraine headaches with aura, and other conditions well summarized by Lam and Zaenglein.[18]

VTE risk is the highest during the first year of treatment, at which time it is approximately 6 to 8 times higher than in untreated age-matched controls.[22] Risk is increased in diabetics, smokers,

Table 1
Combined Oral Contraceptives approved by the FDA for the treatment of acne

Estrostep	Ethinyl estradiol 20 µg/ norethindrone acetate 1 mg
Ortho Tri-Cyclen	Ethinyl estradiol 35 µg/ norgestimate 0.180 mg
Yaz	Ethinyl estradiol 30 µg/ drospirenone 3 mg
Beyaz	Ethinyl estradiol 20 µg/ drospirenone 3 mg/ levomefolic acid 400 µg

those with high body mass index, and during times of immobility and postsurgically.[22,23] There are also many uncommon causes for genetic thrombophilia that increase the risk of VTEs, but these are often first diagnosed when a young woman on COCs experiences her first VTE.[18]

Increased risk of both breast and ovarian cancer has been suggested in the literature. However, the risk is marginal and controversial.[24] In a meta-analysis of 54 studies, there was a relative risk for breast cancer of 1.24.[25] Another study found no difference between users and nonusers.[26] For both breast and ovarian cancer, the relative risk returned to baseline after 10 years of nonuse.[25,27] Confounding the data are the facts that earlier analyses were performed with high-dose EE pills, and that the increased incidence of human papilloma virus seen in COC users may predispose patients to higher risk of cervical cancer.[28,29]

Spironolactone

Spironolactone is a highly effective treatment for women with acne. Despite not being approved by the FDA for the treatment of acne, it is commonly used for acne and other androgen-related disorders in women. Since FDA approval in 1960 it was underused until recently, when it has undergone a renaissance driven by efficacy, safety, and the worldwide effort to avoid the use of antibiotics.

The efficacy and safety of spironolactone has been inadequately studied. The literature is replete with case reports and small case series, often with spironolactone used as an adjunct to other standard agents such as COCs and antibiotics.[30–34] Two small, prospective, placebo-controlled studies showed improvement in acne severity and a reduction of sebum with 50 to 200 mg daily.[30,31] Shaw performed a retrospective chart review of 85 patients treated with spironolactone 50 to 200 mg daily as either monotherapy or adjunctive therapy and found complete or marked improvement in 66%.[32] A study of Asian patients examined spironolactone 200 mg a day for 8 weeks followed by a taper over 20 weeks in 116 women and 23 men.[33] The dropout rate was considerable in the women; the study was discontinued in men because of gynecomastia. All of the 64 women who completed the study reported good to excellent results. In a retrospective study of 110 women using spironolactone monotherapy, 94 patients noted improvement and 61 cleared completely.[35] The authors observed an average total lesion count improvement of 73.1% on the face, and importantly 75.9% and 77.6% on the back, indicating that spironolactone is a useful agent for truncal acne. Although 51 women experienced side effects, only 6 discontinued the drug, implying that the side effects were sufficiently mild compared with the excellent efficacy. In an adjunctive study, spironolactone 100 mg every day and EE 0.03 mg/drospirenone (Yasmin) were added to the existing topical regimen in 27 women with severe papular or nodulocystic acne.[34] Despite extensive disease severity, after 6 months 85% were deemed clear or excellent (≥75%).

Thus, although the available data are encouraging, a large, prospective monotherapy study is lacking. As a result of the small number and size of existing evidence-based data, a Cochrane database review concluded that spironolactone lacked sufficient evidence to support its use in acne.[30] Most recently, Layton and colleagues[36] conducted a hybrid systematic review of all published studies that had evaluated spironolactone efficacy and tolerability in acne. They found 10 usable randomized controlled trials and 21 case series, which were culled in the hope of extracting sufficient data to (1) demonstrate efficacy as monotherapy, (2) aid in identification of characteristics of patients most likely to benefit from its use, and (3) identify the most efficacious and best-tolerated dosing regimen. The authors concluded that these goals were unattainable with our current level of knowledge. The sole efficacy take-home message from the study was that there is very low-quality but highly statistically significant evidence that 200 mg per day is superior to placebo. However, it also showed that the high dose was associated with a greater risk of side effects. Interestingly, despite the "data-penia," expert comments, consensus groups, and current guidelines continue to support the use of spironolactone in women.[1,37,38]

Spironolactone is generally well tolerated, especially at lower doses.[1,36] Common side effects include menstrual irregularities (22%), breast tenderness (17%), breast enlargement, and CNS symptoms (fatigue, dizziness, headache).[27] Although not technically a side effect as spironolactone is a diuretic, diuresis was reported in 29% of patients[27] (**Box 2**).

The most common side effect is menstrual irregularities, seen in approximately 22% of patients.[39] The incidence is greatly decreased by concomitant use of COCs, which have the added advantage of preventing pregnancy and reducing other nuisance side effects such as spotting, weight gain, and mood changes.[34,36,40–42] This pertains even at higher doses of spironolactone whereby disturbances are considerably more common. Hughes and Cunliffe examined menstrual irregularities in 53 women on 200 mg/d and found that

---

Box 2
Spironolactone side effects

Diuresis 29%

Menstrual irregularities 22%

Breast tenderness 17%

Breast enlargement

Fatigue

Dizziness

Headache

---

nearly all women (21 of 24) experienced the side effect on spironolactone alone, whereas only 12 of 23 noted it with COCs.[43]

Hyperkalemia was a considered a theoretic concern because of the potassium-sparing nature of spironolactone diuresis. However, a recent large retrospective database review was performed on women between 18 and 45 years on spironolactone for acne.[44] Only 0.75% (13 of 1802) of samples were elevated and 6 of those retested as normal; these results are similar to those in age-matched controls. The authors concluded that testing potassium in young healthy women taking spironolactone for acne is unnecessary. Layton and colleagues[36] drew the same conclusion after performing a systematic review of the literature. It is important to recognize that the results of these studies may not be generalizable to older women, patients taking higher doses of drug, and women also taking angiotensin-converting enzyme inhibitors, angiotensin receptor blockers, NSAIDs, and digoxin. In addition, it is prudent to recommend avoidance of high-potassium foods such as low-sodium processed foods and coconut water.[45]

The use of spironolactone in women of childbearing potential is somewhat controversial. At doses far in excess of that used in humans, feminization of a male fetus was demonstrated in animal studies.[1] It is uncertain what implications this may have for humans in whom there are very limited data. Most published recommendations for acne therapy during pregnancy recommend discontinuation of spironolactone as a theoretic concern without supporting data.[46] An exhaustive search of the Internet was unsuccessful in finding a report of fetal malformation or other harm to a human fetus. Recognizing that this medication has been available since the 1960s, absence of a single case report implies that the risk in humans is minimal. However, the theoretic risk warrants at the very least a conversation with the patient and use of COCs if appropriate.

Lastly, a black-box warning was recently added to the package insert for spironolactone recommending that its off-label and unnecessary use be avoided. This instruction was based primarily on animal studies in which doses up to 150 times that used in humans were associated with the development of numerous benign and malignant tumors.[1] The literature does not support this association in humans. A search of the Internet reveals only one case report of 5 women with breast cancer who had taken spironolactone along with other medications.[47] However, 5 subsequent retrospective and longitudinal studies have found no association.[39,48–51] No association between spironolactone use and breast cancer was found in a large retrospective, matched cohort study in the United Kingdom of 1.29 million women after 8.4 patient-years of use.[50] Another retrospective cohort study in Denmark of 2.3 million women (28.8 million person-years) found no association with breast uterine, cervical, or ovarian cancers.[51]

ISOTRETINOIN

Approved by the FDA in 1982, isotretinoin recently celebrated its 36th birthday and is still recognized as the most effective acne medication available. In addition, it is unique among acne therapies in that it has the potential to not just treat acne but to eradicate it. When a complete course is taken, approximately 80% of patients will remain free from disease; interestingly, the explanation for this permanent remission evades us.[52]

Isotretinoin efficacy hinges on its ability to affect all of the major pathophysiologic factors of acne. Isotretinoin produces a dramatic reduction in sebum production—90%—in only 6 weeks.[53] It normalizes follicular hyperkeratinization, indirectly reduces *Propionibacterium acnes* colonization, and has anti-inflammatory properties. Clinically this translates into decreased acne lesions and acne scarring along with improvement in psychological symptoms resulting from acne, most notably depression and anxiety.[53–57]

When used for severe acne, isotretinoin therapy is generally initiated with a dose of 0.5 to 1.0 mg/kg/d. Thereafter, the dose is increased toward 1.0 mg/kg/d as tolerated by the patient.[54,58] Although counterintuitive, more severely affected patients may require lower doses with or without concomitant oral corticosteroids to prevent significant flare and increased risk of scarring, what has been termed pseudoacne fulminans.[59] Virtually any dose of isotretinoin will result in short-term clinical improvement, but a remission-free state is the goal. To this end, most authors recommend that a target cumulative dose of 120 to 150 mg/kg is appropriate, although this is not universal.[1] Lower cumulative doses of 0.5 mg/kg were shown to be associated with a higher relapse rate and higher retreatment rate than 1.0 mg/kg.[54,56,58] In other studies, relapse rate was higher in patients dosed with a cumulative dose of less than 120 mg/kg compared with those treated with greater than 120 mg/kg.[54,60] One group suggested that the therapeutic benefits plateau beyond 150 mg/kg cumulative dose[60] while another found that cumulative doses higher than 220 mg/kg were associated with lower relapse rates.[61] Relapse rates are higher in patients treated in their early teens.[62] The cause of this finding is unknown.

In moderate acne, many studies have suggested that lower doses (0.25–0.4 mg/kg/d) and lower cumulative doses are comparable with higher-dose regimens used in severe acne.[63–66] In addition, at lower doses tolerability and patient satisfaction were increased.[63–65] Unlike what was seen in severe acne, low-dose relapse rates in moderate acne were similar to those seen with conventional dosing.[65,66]

Isotretinoin is highly lipophilic and absorption is markedly decreased when taken on an empty stomach.[67–69] Patients should be instructed to take it with meals, preferably one high in fat. A newer branded formulation, isotretinoin-Lidose, uses lipids to encase the medication and is less food-dependent.[69]

The considerable benefits of isotretinoin must be weighed against its risks, both real and perceived. Although adverse events are common, occurring in virtually all patients, they are largely composed of transient nuisance side effects that spontaneously resolve with discontinuation. To a large extent, patient expectation of side effects gleaned from friends and the Internet far exceed reality. However, there are some significant issues and some speculative adverse events that have been extensively reviewed in publications.[70,71] The most common side effects mimic symptoms of hypervitaminosis A and include dry lips, dry eyes, and musculoskeletal complaints.

One putative side effect that gained considerable momentum on the Internet is mood alterations including anxiety and depression. It is certainly the most common concern of patients and patients' parents when starting isotretinoin. These side effects have been uncommonly reported in case studies.[72,73] When attempting to assess the risk of such events, it is important to recognize the high baseline occurrence of anxiety, depression, and suicidal ideation/suicide in the adolescent and young adult population. According to statistics from the National Institutes of Health, major depression is more common in 18- to 25-

year-olds than in any other age group[74] and the Centers for Disease Control and Prevention reports that suicide is the third most common cause of death in adolescence, resulting in 11% of deaths.[75] Not surprisingly, then, multiple studies have failed to find a causative association between isotretinoin and depression on a population basis[76–81]; rather, many have found no change or even an improvement in psychological functioning following successful isotretinoin treatment.[57,76–84] Perhaps the answer lies in several studies from across the world that have found significant associations between acne and depression, mental health problems, and suicide.[85–87]

The most recent speculative association is between isotretinoin and inflammatory bowel disease (IBD), which comprises both ulcerative colitis (UC) and Crohn's disease (CD). Two studies suggested a potential association[88,89] but more recent studies have found no relationship.[90–93] This has been supported by guidelines working groups and the American Academy of Dermatology position paper on isotretinoin.[1,94] Interestingly there is no evidence that isotretinoin use in patients with existing UC/CD worsens disease severity or prognosis.

The teratogenic effects of isotretinoin are well documented. Following the initial launch of the drug in 1982 there were many reports of congenital malformations, and the first of 3 risk management programs was implemented.[95] Each iteration has been more restrictive but no more effective in preventing the approximately 150 exposed pregnancies that occur yearly.[96,97] Our current risk management program, iPLEDGE, was introduced in 2006 and is the most stringent thus far. Women of childbearing potential are required to abstain or to use 2 forms of contraception, and must have a negative pregnancy test before each refill. In a recent study, nearly one-third of women of childbearing potential admitted to noncompliance with the iPLEDGE contraceptive regulations.[97] These data highlight the importance of a frank and thorough discussion of birth control with all patients.

SUMMARY

Available pharmacologic actives for the treatment of acne have changed little in the past decade. The biggest changes have been in our recognition of the need for us to practice better antibiotic stewardship and our search for clinical options. Key in this quest is our recognition that acute therapy, especially when acne is moderate to severe, may bear little resemblance to long-term maintenance therapy in the same patient. No longer are antibiotics considered a long-term treatment option, and this has resulted in renewed interest in existing alternative therapies and the importance of maintenance and combination therapy. Reaffirmation of the unique benefits of benzoyl peroxide and topical retinoids, establishing the usefulness and safety of spironolactone, highlighting the efficacy and safety of anti-inflammatory-dose doxycycline, and emphasizing the importance of early intervention with isotretinoin are current important trends.

REFERENCES

1. Zaenglein A, Pathy A, Schlosser B, et al. Guidelines of care for the treatment of acne vulgaris. J Am Acad Dermatol 2016;74(5):945–73.
2. Dreno B, Layton A, Zouboulis C, et al. Adult female acne: a new paradigm. J Eur Acad Dermatol Venereol 2013;27(9):1063–70.
3. Thiboutot D. Hormones and acne: pathophysiology, clinical evaluation and therapies. Semin Cutan Med Surg 2001;20(3):419–28.
4. Thiboutot D. Acne: hormonal concepts and therapy. Clin Dermatol 2004;22(5):419–28.
5. Thiboutot D. Endocrinological evaluation and hormonal therapy for women with difficult acne. J Eur Acad Dermatol Venereol 2001;15(Suppl 3):57–61.
6. Arowojolu O, Gallo M, Lopez L, et al. Combined oral contraceptive pills for treatment of acne. Cochrane Database Syst Rev 2012;(6):CD004425.
7. Arrington E, Patel N, Gerancher K, et al. Combined oral contraceptives for the treatment of acne: a practical guide. Cutis 2012;90(2):83–90.
8. Kurokawa I, Danby F, Ju Q, et al. New developments in our understanding of acne pathogenesis and treatment. Exp Dermatol 2009;18:821–32.
9. Thiboutot D, Gilliland K, Light J, et al. Androgen metabolism in sebaceous glands from subjects with and without acne. Arch Dermatol 1999;135:1041–5.
10. Davtyan C. Four generations of progestins in oral contraceptives. Proceedings of UCLA Healthcare 2012. p. 16. Available at: www.med.ucla.edu/modules/xfsection/download.php?fileid=638. Accessed September 15, 2018.
11. Lucky A, Koltun W, Thiboutot D, et al. A combined oral contraceptive containing 3-mg drospirenone/20-microg ethinyl estradiol in the treatment of acne vulgaris: a randomized, double-blind, placebo-controlled study evaluating lesion counts and participant self-assessment. Cutis 2008;82:143–50.
12. Maloney J, Dietze P, Watson D, et al. Treatment of acne using a 3-milligram drospirenone/20-microgram ethinyl estradiol oral contraceptive administered in a 24/4 regimen: a randomized controlled trial. Obstet Gynecol 2008;112:773–81.
13. Maloney J, Dietze P, Watson D, et al. A randomized controlled trial of a low-dose combined oral contraceptive containing 3 mg drospirenone plus 20 microg ethinylestradiol in the treatment of acne vulgaris: lesion counts, investigator ratings and subject self-assessment. J Drugs Dermatol 2009;8:837–44.
14. Plewig G, Cunliffe W, Binder N, et al. Efficacy of an oral contraceptive containing EE 0.03 mg and CMA 2 mg (Belara) in moderate acne resolution: a randomized, double-blind, placebo-controlled phase III trial. Contraception 2009;80:25–33.
15. Koltun W, Lucky A, Thiboutot D, et al. Efficacy and safety of 3 mg drospirenone/20 mcg ethinylestradiol oral contraceptive administered in 24/4 regimen in the treatment of acne vulgaris: a randomized, double-blind, placebo-controlled trial. Contraception 2008;77:249–56.
16. Koltun W, Maloney J, Marr J, et al. Treatment of moderate acne vulgaris using a combined oral contraceptive containing ethinylestradiol 20 µg plus drospirenone 3 mg administered in a 24/4 regimen: a pooled analysis. Eur J Obstet Gynecol Reprod Biol 2011;155:171–5.
17. Jaisamrarn U, Chaovisitsaree S, Angsuwathana S. A comparison of multiphasic oral contraceptives containing norgestimate or desogestrel in acne treatment: a randomized trial. Contraception 2014;90:535–41.
18. Lam C, Zaenglein A. Contraceptive use in acne. Clin Dermatol 2014;32(4):502–15.
19. Beral V, Hermon C, Kay C, et al. Mortality associated with oral contraceptive use: 25 year follow up of cohort of 46,000 women from Royal College of General Practitioners: oral contraception study. BMJ 1999;318:96–100.
20. George R, Clarke S, Thiboutot D. Hormonal therapy for acne. Semin Cutan Med Surg 2008;27:188–96.
21. Kim G, Michaels B. Post-adolescent acne in women: more common and more clinical considerations. J Drugs Dermatol 2012;11:708–13.
22. Rott H. Thrombotic risks of oral contraceptives. Curr Opin Obstet Gynecol 2012;24:235–40.
23. Lidegaard O, Edstrom B, Keriner S. Oral contraceptives and venous thromboembolism: a five-year national case-control study. Contraception 2002;65:187–96.
24. Cibula D, Gompel A, Mueck A, et al. Hormonal contraception and risk of cancer. Hum Reprod Update 2010;16:631–50.
25. Collaborative Group on Hormonal Factors in Breast Cancer. Breast cancer and hormonal contraceptives: collaborative reanalysis of individual data on 53,297 women with breast cancer and 100,239 women without breast cancer from 5 epidemiological studies. Lancet 1996;247:1713–27.

26. Marchbanks P, McDonald J, Wilson H, et al. Oral contraceptives and the risk of breast cancer. N Engl J Med 2002;346:2025–32.

27. Appleby P, Beral V, Berrington de Gonzalez A, et al. Cervical cancer and hormonal contraceptives: Collaborative reanalysis of individual data for 16,573 women with cervical cancer and 35,509 women without cervical cancer from 24 epidemiological studies. Lancet 2007;370:1609–21.

28. Drife J. The contraceptive pill and breast cancer in young women. BMJ 1989;298:1269–70.

29. Sasieni P. Cervical cancer prevention and hormonal contraception. Lancet 2007;370:1591–2.

30. Muhlemann M, Carter G, Cream J, et al. Oral spironolactone: an effective treatment for acne vulgaris in women. Br J Dermatol 1986;115:227–32.

31. Goodfellow A, Alaghband-Zadeh J, Carter G, et al. Oral spironolactone improves acne vulgaris and reduces sebum excretion. Br J Dermatol 1984;111: 209–14.

32. Shaw J. Low-dose adjunctive spironolactone in the treatment of acne in women: a retrospective analysis of 85 consecutively treated patients. J Am Acad Dermatol 2000;43:498–502.

33. Sato K, Matsumoto D, Lizuka F, et al. Anti-androgenic therapy using oral spironolactone for acne vulgaris in Asians. Aesthetic Plast Surg 2006;30:689–94.

34. Krunic A, Ciurea A, Scheman A. Efficacy and tolerance of acne treatment using both spironolactone and a combined contraceptive containing drospirenone. J Am Acad Dermatol 2008;58:60–2.

35. Charny J, Choi J, James W. Spironolactone for the treatment of acne in women, a retrospective study of 110 patients. Int J Womens Dermatol 2017;33: 111–5.

36. Layton A, Eady E, Whitehouse H. Oral spironolactone for acne vulgaris in adult women: a hybrid systematic review. Am J Clin Dermatol 2017;18(2): 169–91.

37. Del Rosso J, Harper J, Graber E, et al. Status report from the American Acne and Rosacea Society on medical management of acne in adult women, part 1: overview, clinical characteristics and laboratory evaluation. Cutis 2015;96:236–41.

38. Gollnick H, Bettoli V, Lambert J, et al. A consensus-based practical and daily guide for the treatment of acne patients. J Eur Acad Dermatol Venereol 2016; 30:1480–90.

39. Shaw J, White L. Long-term safety of spironolactone in acne: results of an 8-year followup study. J Cutan Med Surg 2002;6:541–5.

40. Kim G, Del Rosso J. Oral spironolactone in post-teenage female patients with acne vulgaris: practical considerations for the clinician based on current data and clinical experience. J Clin Aesthet Dermatol 2012;5:37–50.

41. Shaw J. Spironolactone in dermatologic therapy. J Am Acad Dermatol 1991;24:236–43.

42. Friedman AJ. Spironolactone for adult female acne. Cutis 2015;96:216–7.

43. Hughes B, Cunliffe W. Tolerance of spironolactone. Br J Dermatol 1988;118:687–91.

44. Plovanich M, Weng Q, Mostaghimi A. Low usefulness of potassium monitoring among healthy young women taking spironolactone for acne. JAMA Dermatol 2015;151:941–4.

45. Zeichner J. Evaluating and treating the adult female patient with acne. J Drugs Dermatol 2013;12: 1416–27.

46. Awan S, Lu J. Management of severe acne during pregnancy: a case report and review of the literature. Int J Women's Dermatol 2017;3:145–50.

47. Loube S, Quirk R. Letter: breast cancer associated with administration of spironolactone. Lancet 1975; 1:1428–9.

48. Danielson D, Jick H, Hunter J, et al. Nonestrogenic drugs and breast cancer. Am J Epidemiol 1982; 116:329–32.

49. Friedman G, Ury H. Initial screening for carcinogenicity of commonly used drugs. J Natl Cancer Inst 1980;65:723–33.

50. Mackenzie I, Macdonald T, Thompson A, et al. Spironolactone and risk of incident breast cancer in women older than 55 years: retrospective, matched cohort study. BMJ 2012;345:e4445.

51. Biggar R, Anderson E, Wohlfahrt J, et al. Spironolactone use and the risk of breast and gynecologic cancers. Cancer Epidemiol 2013;37:870–5.

52. Dispenza M, Wolpert E, Gilliland K. Systemic isotretinoin therapy normalizes exaggerated TLR-2 mediated innate immune responses in acne patients. J Invest Dermatol 2012;132(9):2198–205.

53. Layton A. The use of isotretinoin in acne. Dermato-Endocrinol 2009;1(3):162–9.

54. Layton A, Knaggs H, Taylor J, et al. Isotretinoin for acne vulgaris—10 years later: a safe and successful treatment. Br J Dermatol 1993;129:292–6.

55. Lehucher-Ceyrac D, Weber-Buisset M. Isotretinoin and acne in practice: a prospective analysis of 188 cases over 9 years. Dermatology 1993;186: 123–8.

56. Peck G, Olsen TG, Butkus D, et al. Isotretinoin versus placebo in the treatment of cystic acne. A randomized double-blind study. J Am Acad Dermatol 1982;6:735–45.

57. Rubinow D, Peck G, Squillace K, et al. Reduced anxiety and depression in cystic acne patients after successful treatment with oral isotretinoin. J Am Acad Dermatol 1987;17:25–32.

58. Strauss J, Rapini R, Shalita A, et al. Isotretinoin therapy for acne: results of a multicenter dose-response study. J Am Acad Dermatol 1984;10:490–6.

59. Greywal T, Zaenglein A, Baldwin H, et al. Evidence-based recommendations for the management of acne fulminans and its variants. J Am Acad Dermatol 2017;77(1):109–17.

60. Lehucher-Ceyrac D, de La Salmoniere P, Chastang C, et al. Predictive factors for failure of isotretinoin treatment in acne patients: results from a cohort of 237 patients. Dermatology 1999;198:278–83.

61. Blasiak R, Stamey C, Burkhart C, et al. High-dose isotretinoin treatment and the rate of retrial, relapse and adverse effects in patients with acne vulgaris. JAMA Dermatol 2013;149:1392–8.

62. Liu A, Yang D, Gerhardstein P, et al. Relapse of acne following isotretinoin treatment: a retrospective study of 405 patients. J Drugs Dermatol 2008;7:963–6.

63. Amichai B, Shemer A, Grunwald M. Low-dose isotretinoin in the treatment of acne vulgaris. J Am Acad Dermatol 2006;54:644–6.

64. Agarwal U, Besarwal R, Bhola K. Oral isotretinoin in different dose regimens for acne vulgaris: a randomized comparative trial. Indian J Dermatol Venereol Leprol 2011;77:688–94.

65. Akman A, Durusoy C, Senturk M, et al. Treatment of acne with intermittent and conventional isotretinoin: a randomized, controlled multicenter study. Arch Dermatol Res 2007;299:467–73.

66. Borghi A, Mantovani L, Minghetti S, et al. Low-cumulative dose isotretinoin treatment in mild-to-moderate acne: efficacy in achieving stable remission. J Eur Acad Dermatol Venereol 2011;25:1094–8.

67. Strauss J, Leyden J, Lucky A, et al. A randomized trial of the efficacy of a new micronized formulation versus a standard formulation of isotretinoin in patients with severe recalcitrant nodular acne. J Am Acad Dermatol 2001;45:187–95.

68. Strauss J, Leyden J, Lucky A, et al. Safety of a new micronized formulation of isotretinoin in patients with severe recalcitrant nodular acne: a randomized trial comparing micronized isotretinoin with standard isotretinoin. J Am Acad Dermatol 2001;45:196–207.

69. Webster G, Leyden J, Gross J. Comparative pharmacokinetic profiles of a novel isotretinoin formulation (isotretinoin-Lidose) and the innovator isotretinoin formulation: a randomized, 4-treatment, crossover study. J Am Acad Dermatol 2013;69:762–7.

70. Strauss J, Krowchuk D, Leyden J, et al. Guidelines of care for acne vulgaris management. J Am Acad Dermatol 2007;56:651–63.

71. Vallerand I, Lewinson R, Farris M, et al. Efficacy and adverse effects of oral isotretinoin for acne: a systematic review. Br J Dermatol 2018;178(1):76–85.

72. Sundstrom A, Alfredsson L, Sjolin-Forsberg G, et al. Association of suicide attempts with acne and treatment with isotretinoin: retrospective Swedish cohort study. BMJ 2010;341:c5812.

73. Marqueling A, Zane L. Depression and suicidal behavior in acne patients treated with isotretinoin: a systematic review. Semin Cutan Med Surg 2005;24:92–102.

74. Available at: www.ninh.nih.gov/health/statistics/major-depression.shtml. Accessed September 12, 2018.

75. Available at: www.cdc.gov/nchs/products/databriefs/db37.pdf. Accessed September 12, 2018.

76. Bozdag K, Gulseren S, Guven F, et al. Evaluation of depressive symptoms in acne patients treated with isotretinoin. J Dermatol Treat 2009;20:293–6.

77. Chia C, Lane W, Chibnall J, et al. Isotretinoin therapy and mood changes in adolescents with moderate to severe acne: a cohort study. Arch Dermatol 2001;141:557–60.

78. Cohen J, Adams S, Patten S. No association found between patients receiving isotretinoin for acne and the development of depression in a Canadian prospective cohort. Can J Clin Pharmacol 2007;14:e227–33.

79. Jick S, Kremers H, Vasilakis-Scaramozza C. Isotretinoin use and risk of depression, psychotic symptoms, suicide and attempted suicide. Arch Dermatol 2000;136:1231–6.

80. Nevoralova Z, Dvorakova D. Mood changes, depression and suicide risk during isotretinoin treatment: a prospective study. Int J Dermatol 2013;52:163–8.

81. Rehn L, Meririnne E, Hook-Nikanne J, et al. Depressive symptoms and suicidal ideation during isotretinoin treatment: a 12-week follow-up study of male Finnish military conscripts. J Eur Acad Dermatol Venereol 2009;23:1294–7.

82. Hull S, Cunliffe W, Hughes B. Treatment of the depressed and dysmorphophobic acne patient. Clin Exp Dermatol 1991;16:210–1.

83. Myhill J, Leichtman S, Burnett J. Self-esteem and social assertiveness in patients receiving isotretinoin treatment for cystic acne. Cutis 1988;41:171–3.

84. Ormerod A, Thind C, Rice S, et al. Influence of isotretinoin on hippocampal based learning in human subjects. Psychopharmacology 2012;221:667–74.

85. Halvorsen J, Stern R, Dalgard F. Suicidal ideation, mental health problems and social impairment are increased in adolescents with acne: a population-based study. J Invest Dermatol 2011;131(2):363070.

86. Rose C, Spelman L, Oziemski M. Isotretinoin and mental health in adolescents: Australian consensus. Australas J Dermatol 2014;55(2):162–7.

87. Yang Y, Tu H, Hong C. Female gender and acne disease are jointly and independently associated with the risk of major depression and suicide: a national population-based study. Biomed Res Int 2014;2014:504279.

88. Crockett S, Gulati A, Sandler R, et al. A causal association between isotretinoin and inflammatory bowel disease has yet to be established. Am J Gastroenterol 2009;104:2387–93.

89. Dubeau M, Iacucci M, Beck P. Drug-induced inflammatory bowel disease and IBD-like conditions. Inflamm Bowel Dis 2013;19:445–56.

90. Alhusayen R, Juurlink D, Mamdani M, et al. Isotretinoin use and the risk of inflammatory bowel disease: a population-based cohort study. J Invest Dermatol 2013;133:907–12.

91. Etminan M, Bird S, Delaney J, et al. Isotretinoin and risk for inflammatory bowel disease: a nested case-control study and meta-analysis of published and unpublished data. JAMA Dermatol 2013;149:216–20.

92. Rashtak S, Khaleghi S, Pittelkow M, et al. Isotretinoin exposure and risk of inflammatory bowel disease. JAMA Dermatol 2014;150:1322–6.

93. Bernstein C, Nugent Z, Longobardi T, et al. Isotretinoin is not associated with inflammatory bowel disease: a population-based case-control study. Am J Gastroenterol 2009;104:2774–8.

94. American Academy of Dermatology website. Position statement on isotretinoin. Available at: www.aad.org/Forms/Policies/Uploads/PS/PS-isotretinoin.pdf. Accessed September 12, 2018.

95. Dai W, LaBraico J, Stern R. Epidemiology of isotretinoin exposure during pregnancy. J Am Acad Dermatol 1992;26:599–606.

96. Shin J, Cheetham T, Wong L, et al. The impact of the iPLEDGE program on isotretinoin fetal exposure in an integrative health care system. J Am Acad Dermatol 2011;65:1117–25.

97. Collins M, Moreau J, Opel D, et al. Compliance with pregnancy prevention measures during isotretinoin therapy. J Am Acad Dermatol 2014;70:55–9.

What's New in Atopic Dermatitis

Yael Renert-Yuval, MD[a], Emma Guttman-Yassky, MD, PhD[b],*

KEYWORDS

- Atopic dermatitis • Crisaborole • Dupiluamb • Tralokinumab • Lebrikizumab • Fezakinumab
- GBR 830 • JAK inhibitors

KEY POINTS

- Atopic dermatitis (AD) is increasingly common, and it lacked effective, safe, long-lasting treatments for many years.
- Recently, novel understandings of AD pathogenesis revealed AD has a complex, heterogeneous molecular fingerprint among different age groups and ethnicities, with a dominant helper T-cell $(T_H)2/T_H22$ skewing and variable T_H17/T_H1 overexpression.
- These findings led to rapid developments of numerous agents studied in clinical trials for AD. Few are already approved and available for clinical use.
- New topical agents for AD include phosphodiesterase 4 inhibitor, JAK (Januse kinase) inhibitors, and commensal bacteria.
- Systemic agents include targeted monoclonal antibodies, antagonizing $T_H2/T_H22/T_H17$-related cytokines, and broad-acting systemic therapeutics, including JAK inhibitors and histamine 4 receptor antihistamines.

INTRODUCTION

Atopic dermatitis (AD), perhaps the most common inflammatory skin disease, with an increasing prevalence worldwide, is characterized by chronic symptoms of eczema and pruritus.[1] The quality of life of AD patients is significantly impaired, with higher prevalence of sleep disturbances, anxiety, depression, and even suicidal ideation compared with the general population.[2] Of AD patients, up to 20% are classified as moderate to severe by various clinical measurements, with the SCOring Atopic Dermatitis (SCORAD), the Eczema Area and Severity Index (EASI), and the Investigator Global Assessment (IGA) most commonly used.[3] Current therapeutics for extensive AD are lacking and consist of broad, nonspecific treatments, providing symptomatic and temporary relief with significant and prevalent adverse-effects.[1,4,5]

In the past few years, extensive research shed light on the pathogenesis of the disease, allowing better understanding of the immune dysregulations causing the clinical outcome of AD. As was the case for psoriasis, which represents the best

Disclosure Statement: E. Guttman-Yassky received board membership from Sanofi Aventis, Regeneron, Stiefel/GlaxoSmithKline, MedImmune, Celgene, Anacor, Leo Pharma, AnaptysBio, Celsus, Dermira, Galderma, Novartis, Pfizer, Vitae, Glenmark, AbbVie, and Asana Biosciences and consultancy fees from Regeneron, Sanofi Aventis, MedImmune, Celgene, Stiefel/GlaxoSmithKline, Celsus, BMS, Amgen, Drais, AbbVie, Anacor, AnaptysBio, Dermira, Galderma, Leo Pharma, Novartis, Pfizer, Vitae, Mitsubishi Tanabe, Eli Lilly, Glenmark, and Asana Biosciences; her institution received grants from Regeneron, Celgene, BMS, Janssen, Dermira, Leo Pharma, Merck, Novartis, and UCB for other works. Y. Renert-Yuval received payment for lectures from Sanofi Israel.
[a] Department of Dermatology, Hadassah-Hebrew University Medical Center, Hadassah Ein-Kerem Medical Center, POB13000, Jerusalem, Israel; [b] Department of Dermatology, Laboratory for Inflammatory Skin Diseases, Icahn School of Medicine at Mount Sinai, 5 East 98th Street, New York, NY 10029, USA
* Corresponding author. Department of Dermatology, Icahn School of Medicine at Mount Sinai Medical Center, 5 East 98th Street, New York, NY 10029.
E-mail address: Emma.Guttman@mountsinai.org

Dermatol Clin 37 (2019) 205–213
https://doi.org/10.1016/j.det.2018.12.007

derm.theclinics.com

existing model for translational studies derma-tology, this translational revolution led to the development of numerous new treatment methods for AD.[6]

It is difficult to write a "what is new in AD" review because this field is so rapidly evolving. This article reviews the new era of AD, with the latest discoveries in the pathogenesis of AD, leading to the developments of novel topical as well as systemic—both broad-acting and specific—agents for the disease.

PATHOPHYSIOLOGY

Traditionally, AD was considered a helper T-cell (T_H)2/T_H1 disease, with T_H2 activation characterizing acute lesions and primarily T_H1 skewing in chronic lesions.[7] Recent extensive translational investigations have shown, however, that AD is strongly T_H2/T_H22 centered throughout its course, with some T_H1 and TH_{17} overexpression.[7,8] The onset of acute AD skin lesions is characterized by large increases in T_H2/T_H22-related cytokines and chemokines and some T_H17-related signals.[9] Later in the disease, intensification of these axes as well as T_H1 augmentation orchestrates the chronic phenotype.[7,10]

The pathogenic contribution of each pathway to the clinical presentation of AD across its various disease phenotypes is still not fully determined, because AD encompasses different clinical subtypes and molecular phenotypes.[9,11–13] AD subtypes that were characterized immunologically so far as relatively T_H17-dominant include the Asian-origin AD, intrinsic AD (approximately 20% of the patients, typically having normal serum IgE levels and lacking personal or familial atopy),[12] and pediatric AD.[11–14] It is important to point out that despite having T_H17-related up-regulations, these AD subtypes still have robust T_H2/T_H22 activation, differing them from psoriasis, which is primarily T_H17 skewed. Recently, African Americans with AD were shown largely T_H2 and T_H22 skewed, lacking T_H1 activation.[15] A lack of T_H1 activation has also been seen in pediatric AD, perhaps arguing against a pathogenic role for this axis in AD.[13,16]

The identification of the inflammatory pathways underlying AD has led to the development and testing of a new set of targeted and broad therapeutics for AD.

Due to the central role of T_H2 activation in the disease, anti-T_H2 drugs were developed early, and the first monoclonal antibody to be approved for the treatment of moderate-to-severe AD, dupilumab, is an antagonist of this pathway.[17–20]

Because AD has a complex immune fingerprint, however, with diverse phenotypic subtypes among different subpopulations and a response of EASI-90 (90% improvement) to dupilumab seen in approximately 30% of patients,[18] other therapeutic targets, in the T_H22 and T_H17 axes, as well as broad-acting agents, are also being studied.

TOPICAL TREATMENTS

Topical therapy is an important component of AD care, even in these times of newly introduced highly effective systemic drugs. The topical treatment is used for barrier repair and delivery of anti-inflammatory compounds, and the mainstay of disease management includes generous use of emollients and moisturizers. For many years, the only active topical agents used as an anti-inflammatory were topical corticosteroids and calcineurin inhibitors. As the treatment paradigm of AD expands, however, new topical drugs are also introduced.

The first drug to be licensed, crisaborole, is a phosphodiesterase (PDE) 4 antagonist. In AD, elevated PDE activity was found compared with normal skin.[21,22] PDE hydrolyzes cyclic adenosine monophosphate (cAMP) and results in up-regulation of inflammatory mediators. PDE antagonism acts in a broad, nonspecific mechanism, because it elevates intracellular cAMP; thus, downstream inhibition of numerous proinflammatory factors ensues.[21]

Crisaborole 2% topical ointment is indicated in adults and children over 2 years of age with mild-to-moderate AD. The ointment showed statistically significant efficacy, with 51.7% and 48.5% of patients achieving Investigator's Static Global Assessment scores of clear or almost clear, respectively, during phase III clinical trials.[23] Crisaborole 2% also improved other AD symptoms, including pruritus,[23] and showed tolerability in sensitive anatomic skin locations, including the face/hairline, genitalia, and intertriginous areas, where treatment with topical corticosteroids is often avoided due to adverse effects.[24] Overall, the ointment was well tolerated with limited adverse events, most commonly application-site pain, burning, or stinging.[23,24]

Another promising group of topical agents, now in clinical trials for AD, are the Janus kinase (JAK) inhibitors. The JAKs, a family of tyrosine kinases (TYKs), including JAK1, JAK2, JAK3, and TYK2, phosphorylate the intracellular domain of several cytokine receptors to facilitate the attachment and stimulation of the signal transducer and activator of transcription (STAT), which then enters the nucleus and effects transcription.[25] As discussed later, these are being tested as systemic treatment of AD, but topical formulations had also shown efficacy in phase II trials. In a 4-week clinical trial of tofacitinib, the ointment showed robust and significantly greater efficacy versus placebo.[26] Nevertheless, topical tofacitinib for AD has not progressed past phase II trials. JTE-032, a topical JAK inhibitor that antagonizes all 4 receptor-associated kinases, markedly and rapidly improved clinical signs and symptoms in 327 Japanese adult AD patients, with a favorable safety profile.[27] Other topical JAKs are being investigated in clinical trials in the pediatric population and adults, including topical ruxolitinib in phosphate cream (ClinicalTrials.gov: NCT03257644 and NCT03011892). A dual SYK/JAK inhibitor, cerdulatinib, is also anticipated to be tested for AD.

A different possible topical therapy relies on another aspect of AD pathophysiology, the disrupted skin microbiome of AD patients. During flares, the diversity of the bacteria that normally reside on the skin is reduced, and there is a shift toward Staphylococcus aureus colonization.[28] S aureus has an important pathogenic role in AD, because it perpetuates the inflammation, specifically T_H2-related, and further compromises skin barrier. Autologous microbiome transplant in 1 study and application of commensal gram-negative bacteria in another led to decreased colonization of S aureus, with clinical improvement and reduced used of topical corticosteroids in the second study.[28,29]

These data suggest newer topical nonsteroidal agents may play an important role as primary therapy or as adjunctive steroid-sparing therapy for AD in the near future and will expand the current limited variety of topical therapy given for AD.

SYSTEMIC TARGETED AGENTS—HELPER T-CELL 2 ANTAGONISTS
Dupilumab, Tralokinumab, and Lebrikizumab

Cytokine-targeted drugs currently are an important therapeutic tool in dermatology, and because AD is largely T_H2/T_H22 centered, antagonizing these axes have strong rationale for AD treatment.

Dupilumab is a fully human monoclonal antibody inhibiting both interleukin (IL)-4 and IL-13 signaling, by blocking their common IL-4 receptor-α (IL-4Rα). Due to the key pathogenic role IL-4 and IL-13 play as initiators and drivers of the T_H2 axis, blocking both cytokines has strong anti-T_H2 effects. Elevated IL-4/IL-13 levels disrupt skin barrier by inhibiting lipids, tight junctions, and antimicrobial peptide formation; interrupting

keratinocytes differentiation; and initiating and poropogating S aureus colonization.[28,30,31] IL-4/IL-13, therefore, have a major part in perpetuating AD, both molecularly and clinically.

In stage II and III clinical trials of dupilumab versus placebo in AD patients, dupilumab was significantly more effective in all primary and secondary outcome measures.[17–19] Furthermore, recent meta-analyses of these trials,[32,33] including more than 2400 adult AD patients, showed dupilumab was consistently more effective than placebo and had an acceptable, placebo-like safety profile. Only local injection side reactions and conjunctivitis occurred as specific side effects of dupilumab.[32,33] The pathogenesis of this conjunctivitis is yet to be elucidated.[34] Coupled with these clinical score improvements, expression of T_H2-related markers was reduced as were markers of epidermal hyperplasia, immune cells infiltrates in the skin, and T_H17/T_H22 activity. Dupilumab also improved the expression of genes of epidermal differentiation, barrier function, and lipid metabolism and suppressed T_H2-related serum biomarkers.[20]

Except dupilumab, which almost entirely blocks T_H2 activation, there are also exclusive anti–IL-13 agents being investigated for AD: tralokinumab and lebrikizumab, both of which are fully humanized monoclonal antibodies.

Tralokinumab binds 2 different receptors: the heterodimeric receptor, composed of IL-4Rα (targeted by dupilumab) and IL-13Rα1, and the IL-13Rα2 decoy receptor, which results in lower cytokine levels.[35] Tralokinumab is now in phase III clinical trials for asthma and AD (NCT03363854). In asthma, predictive biomarkers for tralokinumab efficacy were serum dipeptidyl peptidase 4 and periostin, which correlate with increased IL-13 activity. The same biomarkers were monitored in the AD phase II clinical trial. In this trial, different doses were studied in 204 AD adult patients with concomitant topical corticosteroids. Here, the highest applied dose of tralokinumab led to significant improvements in clinical scores versus placebo, yet high placebo responses were seen, probably due to concomitant topical corticosteroid application. The drug was overall well tolerated. Similarly to asthma, greater, significant responses were found in the subpopulation with high concentrations of IL-13–related biomarkers, suggesting these markers have predictive value for the efficacy of anti–IL-13 therapy in AD patients.[36]

Lebrikizumab binds the soluble IL-13 at an epitope that strongly overlaps with the binding site of IL-4Rα[37] and is also investigated for asthma as well as for AD (NCT03443024) and other conditions. It was studied in proof-of-concept phase II study on adults with AD in combination with mandatory topical corticosteroids.[38] At 12 weeks, significantly more patients achieved a 50% reduction of the severity score EASI (EASI-50) with lebrikizumab, although pronounced placebo responses were seen, speculatively due to the topical corticosteroid use. It was concluded that protocol-mandated topical corticosteroid limited investigators' ability to fully evaluate lebrikizumab's efficacy in AD. The drug was well tolerated.[38]

These positive data raise the possibility that narrow IL-13 targeting may also be a valid future therapy for AD, and clinical trials investigating these drugs as monotherapy are needed.

Interleukin 31 Blockers

Despite the suggested pivotal role of IL-4/IL-13 in AD, skin lesions of AD are characterized by robust up-regulations of various other T_H2-related cytokines and chemokines, and these too have the potential of being therapeutic targets.[7,9]

Nemolizumab, another monoclonal antibody, antagonizes IL-31 receptor A and thus blocks IL-31 signaling on various cells, including peripheral neurons.[39] IL-31, a T_H2-related cytokine, also known as the itch cytokine, is significantly up-regulated in AD lesions.[40,41] In addition, cytokine levels correlate with disease severity, and up-regulated IL-31 was shown to compromise epidermal-barrier function, perpetuating the well-documented itch-scratch cycle of AD.[40,41] Notwithstanding, despite the possible potential of anti–IL-31 targeting, a phase II randomized, double-blind, placebo-controlled study of nemolizumab for AD showed improvements in clinical scores but did not reach statistical significance. Nemolizumab did significantly decrease pruritus scores and had an overall satisfactory safety profile.[39]

Clinical trials for another anti–IL-31 monoclonal antibody, BMS-981164, were terminated at an early stage (NCT01614756). Thus, the role of IL-31 antagonism in AD treatment is still to be elucidated, because it is not clear if the effects include only symptomatic, antipruritic relief.

Inhibitors of the Thymic Stromal Lymphopoietin–OX40 Axis

The T_H2 pathway also includes the thymic stromal lymphopoietin (TSLP)-OX40 axis, which is speculated to initiate the allergic response and is referred as the master switch of allergic inflammation.[42,43] Through the effects of this axis on dendritic cells, Langerhans cells, and mast cells, T_H2-skewed responses ensues, and CD4$^+$ T-naïve

cells are activated to produce IL-4, IL-13, and IL-5.[43,44] OX40 ligand (OX40L) is downstream to TSLP and was shown to deepen T_H2 polarization and maintain chronic allergic inflammation.[45,46] IL-33 is an amplifier of the TSLP-OX40L axis and was also shown to directly disturb skin barrier in AD by down-regulating FLG expression.[47,48] TSLP, its receptor, OX40L, and IL-33 are significantly up-regulated in lesional AD skin,[47,49] providing another possible therapeutic targets for AD.

Tezepelumab, a monoclonal antibody antagonizing TSLP, failed in a phase II clinical trial for AD (NCT02525094),[50] and MK-8226, a TSLP receptor antagonist (NCT01732510), was terminated due to business reasons. An OX40 antagonist, GBR 830 (NCT02683928), showed efficacy in a phase II clinical trial after 2 intravenous doses. Significantly more GBR 830-treated patients versus placebo achieved EASI-50 after more than 2 months, a long-lasting effect despite the convenient and minimal dosing. The drug was well tolerated.[51] KHK4083, another OX40 inhibitor, is being investigated in a phase I open-label clinical trial for AD in Japan (NCT03096223).[52] An anti–IL-33 monoclonal antibody, ANB020, showed efficacy in a small, proof-of-concept, phase II clinical trial of adult AD patients.[53] Because OX40 and IL-33 inhibitors show promise, future studies are anticipated. TSLP inhibitors may, speculatively, emerge in the future as treatments of very early AD, due to its role in disease onset.

TARGETING HELPER T-CELL 22

In addition to common T_H2 skewing across all AD subtypes, T_H22-related genes are also overexpressed, and the main cytokine in this axis, IL-22, plays a major role in barrier function disruption, by down-regulating terminal differentiation and tight junction products, and promotes epidermal hyperplasia resulting in acanthosis.[54–56] IL-22 is significantly up-regulated in AD lesions and has been correlated to disease severity and clinical response to various AD treatments.[57–63]

An anti–IL-22 antibody, fezakinumab, showed numerical efficacy that did not reach significance in a randomized, double-blind, placebo-controlled trial for AD as a monotherapy.[64] Despite these somewhat disappointing results, subanalyses of only severe AD patients revealed significance response to fezakinumab over placebo.[64] A mechanistic study of fezakinumab showed the drug's effects were stratified depending on baseline IL-22 expression, with molecular response present only in high baseline IL-22 patients, perhaps opening the door to a personalized medicine approach for AD.[65] In addition, similarly to dupilumab, significant down-regulations of multiple immune pathways, including T_H1, T_H2, T_H17, and T_H22, were found in patients with high IL-22 levels treated with fezakinumab .[65] Fezakinumab was well tolerated, and the most common adverse events were viral upper respiratory tract infections.[64]

These data suggest fezakizumab may serve as an agent for severe AD patients or for patients with unsatisfactory response to T_H2 inhibition by dupilumab,[64] yet reliable predictors for drug efficacy still need to be validated in larger, extended studies.

HELPER T-CELL 17/INTERLEUKIN 23 ANTAGONISM

As discussed previously, in addition to the common T_H2/T_H22 overexpression, some AD phenotypes (including Asian AD, intrinsic AD, and pediatric AD) show higher T_H17-related markers expression as well as histologic features that are also seen in psoriasis, which is T_H17/T_H1 driven.[66,67]

IL-23 prompts both T_H17 and T_H22, and, downstream to IL-23, IL-17 with IL-22 stimulates tissue inflammation and barrier defects.[68] In addition, IL-23 is significantly decreased after AD treatments,[57–60,62] providing a rationale for IL-23 antagonism in AD.

Ustekinumab, a monoclonal antibody antagonizing the p40 subunit of IL-23 and IL-12, is highly efficacious for psoriasis.[69] For AD, however, despite several reports of refractory AD responsive to ustekinumab treatment,[70,71] a phase II clinical trial of ustekinumab showed numerical improvements in clinical scores but did not reach statistical significant over placebo.[61]

As for IL-17, the IL-17 family consists of 6 members, IL-17A–F.[72] IL-17A and IL-17F are products of activated lymphocytes, and IL-17E and IL-17C are products of epidermal keratinocytes and other nonimmune cells.[73] Nevertheless, IL-17A and IL-17C share some features, as keratinocytes respond to these cytokines in a similar manner.[73,74] In addition, there is a robust connection between IL-17A and IL-17C, because IL-17A induces IL-17C in keratinocytes, and, in turn, IL-17C can induce IL-17A production in T lymphocytes. This relationship can be viewed as part of the feed-forward mechanism in the epidermis, in which amplification of cellular immune responses results from overexpression of cytokines and chemokines produced by keratinocytes.[75]

IL-17A inhibition by drugs, such as secukinumab, a monoclonal antibody that selectively inhibits IL-17A and is highly efficacious in psoriasis,[76] is being tested for AD in a phase II clinical trial (NCT02594098).

The interest in IL-17C is growing, as overexpression of IL-17C was found in skin lesions of both psoriasis and AD compared with control skin, and, with other data suggesting IL-17C has a pathogenic role as a central mediator of inflammation in both diseases, antagonism of IL-17C seems to be an appealing strategy.[73,74]

A phase I clinical trial of an anti–IL-17C monoclonal antibody, MOR106, showed encouraging clinical results in AD, with approximately 80% of drug-treated patients achieving EASI-50 compared with less than 20% in the placebo group, with a favorable safety profile.[77] This positive yet small, early-phase, proof-of-concept trial necessitates further studies (now recruiting, NCT03568071), preferably in larger cohorts of AD and across different AD phenotypes, to reveal the potential of IL-17C antagonism in subpopulations with higher T_H17 activity.

BROAD-ACTING SYSTEMIC AGENTS

Even though narrow-targeted agents in AD proved that blocking 1 cytokine may have a much broader effect on immune dysregulations, including upstream to the antagonized cytokine, broad-acting agents are another important possible tool in the armamentarium of AD treatments.

Janus Kinase Inhibitors

The JAK-STAT, as discussed previously, mediates T_H2 polarization in addition to a range of other intracellular immune dysregulations.[78] Oral JAK inhibitors are small molecules that block these intracellular signaling and result in a potent, broad, inhibition of various inflammatory pathways as well as antiproliferative activity.[79]

Currently, 3 JAK inhibitors are studied in clinical trials for AD: baricitinib, a JAK 1 and JAK 2 antagonist; upadacitinib, a JAK1 antagonist; and PF-04965842 (abrocitinib), another specific JAK1 inhibitor.

Baricitinib is the first JAK inhibitor to show efficacy in a phase II trial for AD[80] and is now in ongoing phase III trials (NCT03435081). With baricitinib, significantly more patients achieved EASI-50 compared with placebo (61% vs 37%) at 16 weeks, and the proportion of baricitinib-treated patients achieving EASI-50 compared with placebo was significant as early as week 4.[80] The drug was well tolerated, yet more adverse events occurred in the baricitinib-treated group, with headache, increased blood creatine phosphokinase, and nasopharyngitis.[80]

Upadacitinib showed impressive and significant clinical efficacy in a phase II clinical trial for AD. In the upadacitinib group, approximately 50% of patients achieved EASI-90, and the same percentage attained IGA of clear or almost clear skin, with a good safety profile, as presented in the 2018 American Academy of Dermatology meeting (NCT02925117).[81] Peer-reviewed publication is still pending.

A third JAK inhibitor, PF-04965842 (abrocitinib), was also investigated in a phase II clinical trial for AD and showed promising results as assessed by the IGA score at week 12, with responses of up to 45% in drug-treated group compared with 6% in the placebo group.[82] A phase III trial for PF-04965842 is now recruiting (NCT03349060).

Histamine 4 Receptor Antihistamines

Other broad-acting, oral, small molecules, representing an additional promising treatment option for AD, are the histamine 4 receptor (H_4R) antihistamines. Unlike the H_1R-blocking antihistamines that traditionally are used as antipruritic agents, yet with effects in AD patients relying mostly on their sedative properties,[83] H_4R antihistamines have implications relevant to AD pathogenesis. H_4R is highly expressed on keratinocytes in lesional skin of AD patients, and its stimulation promotes keratinocyte proliferation and inhibits their differentiation, impairs skin barrier, and induces pruritus.[84,85] A phase II clinical trial of ZPL-3893787, an H_4R antagonist, is ongoing (NCT02424253).

SUMMARY

Despite a highly prevalent disease, until recently AD lacked effective, safe, long-term treatment options for moderate-to-severe patients. Now, however, it is somewhat challenging to keep up with the extremely rapid pace of developments in AD. Recent data revealing the molecular underpinnings of AD, together with the huge unmet need for efficacious, safe therapies, and vigorous industry interest in developing new medications,[1] led to the current exciting era of numerous therapeutics investigated for the disease. Novel agents—topical and systemic, narrow targeted and broad acting—will be introduced to AD management in the near future and will revolutionize the treatment paradigm of the disease.

REFERENCES

1. Brunner PM, Leung DYM, Guttman-Yassky E. Immunologic, microbial, and epithelial interactions in atopic dermatitis. Ann Allergy Asthma Immunol 2018;120(1):34–41.
2. Ronnstad ATM, Halling-Overgaard AS, Hamann CR, et al. Association of atopic dermatitis with depression, anxiety, and suicidal ideation in children and adults: a systematic review and meta-analysis. J Am Acad Dermatol 2018;79(3):448–56.e30.
3. Wollenberg A, Oranje A, Deleuran M, et al. ETFAD/EADV Eczema task force 2015 position paper on diagnosis and treatment of atopic dermatitis in adult and paediatric patients. J Eur Acad Dermatol Venereol 2016;30(5):729–47.
4. Saeki H, Nakahara T, Tanaka A, et al. Clinical practice guidelines for the management of atopic dermatitis 2016. J Dermatol 2016;43(10):1117–45.
5. Renert-Yuval Y, Guttman-Yassky E. Monoclonal antibodies for the treatment of atopic dermatitis. Curr Opin Allergy Clin Immunol 2018;18(4):356–64.
6. Guttman-Yassky E, Krueger JG, Lebwohl MG. Systemic immune mechanisms in atopic dermatitis and psoriasis with implications for treatment. Exp Dermatol 2018;27(4):409–17.
7. Gittler JK, Shemer A, Suarez-Farinas M, et al. Progressive activation of T(H)2/T(H)22 cytokines and selective epidermal proteins characterizes acute and chronic atopic dermatitis. J Allergy Clin Immunol 2012;130(6):1344–54.
8. Malajian D, Guttman-Yassky E. New pathogenic and therapeutic paradigms in atopic dermatitis. Cytokine 2015;73(2):311–8.
9. Czarnowicki T, Krueger JG, Guttman-Yassky E. Skin barrier and immune dysregulation in atopic dermatitis: an evolving story with important clinical implications. J Allergy Clin Immunol Pract 2014;2(4):371–9 [quiz: 80–1].
10. Thepen T, Langeveld-Wildschut EG, Bihari IC, et al. Biphasic response against aeroallergen in atopic dermatitis showing a switch from an initial TH2 response to a TH1 response in situ: an immunocytochemical study. J Allergy Clin Immunol 1996;97(3):828–37.
11. Noda S, Suarez-Farinas M, Ungar B, et al. The Asian atopic dermatitis phenotype combines features of atopic dermatitis and psoriasis with increased TH17 polarization. J Allergy Clin Immunol 2015;136(5):1254–64.
12. Suarez-Farinas M, Dhingra N, Gittler J, et al. Intrinsic atopic dermatitis shows similar TH2 and higher TH17 immune activation compared with extrinsic atopic dermatitis. J Allergy Clin Immunol 2013;132(2):361–70.
13. Esaki H, Brunner PM, Renert-Yuval Y, et al. Early-onset pediatric atopic dermatitis is TH2 but also TH17 polarized in skin. J Allergy Clin Immunol 2016;138(6):1639–51.
14. Czarnowicki T, Esaki H, Gonzalez J, et al. Early pediatric atopic dermatitis shows only a cutaneous

lymphocyte antigen (CLA)(+) TH2/TH1 cell imbalance, whereas adults acquire CLA(+) TH22/TC22 cell subsets. J Allergy Clin Immunol 2015;136(4): 941–51.e3.

15. Sanyal RD, Pavel AB, Glickman J, et al. Atopic dermatitis in African American patients is TH2/TH22-skewed with TH1/TH17 attenuation. Ann Allergy Asthma Immunol 2018. https://doi.org/10.1016/j.anai.2018.08.024.

16. Czarnowicki T, Esaki H, Gonzalez J, et al. Alterations in B-cell subsets in pediatric patients with early atopic dermatitis. J Allergy Clin Immunol 2017; 140(1):134–44.e9.

17. Thaci D, Simpson EL, Beck LA, et al. Efficacy and safety of dupilumab in adults with moderate-to-severe atopic dermatitis inadequately controlled by topical treatments: a randomised, placebo-controlled, dose-ranging phase 2b trial. Lancet 2016;387(10013):40–52.

18. Simpson EL, Bieber T, Guttman-Yassky E, et al. Two phase 3 trials of dupilumab versus placebo in atopic dermatitis. N Engl J Med 2016;375(24):2335–48.

19. Blauvelt A, de Bruin-Weller M, Gooderham M, et al. Long-term management of moderate-to-severe atopic dermatitis with dupilumab and concomitant topical corticosteroids (LIBERTY AD CHRONOS): a 1-year, randomised, double-blinded, placebo-controlled, phase 3 trial. Lancet 2017;389(10086): 2287–303.

20. Guttman-Yassky E, Bissonnette R, Ungar B, et al. Dupilumab progressively improves systemic and cutaneous abnormalities in atopic dermatitis patients. J Allergy Clin Immunol 2018. https://doi.org/10.1016/j.jaci.2018.08.022.

21. Schafer PH, Parton A, Capone L, et al. Apremilast is a selective PDE4 inhibitor with regulatory effects on innate immunity. Cell Signal 2014;26(9): 2016–29.

22. Jarnagin K, Chanda S, Coronado D, et al. Crisaborole topical ointment, 2%: a nonsteroidal, topical, anti-inflammatory phosphodiesterase 4 inhibitor in clinical development for the treatment of atopic dermatitis. J Drugs Dermatol 2016;15(4):390–6.

23. Paller AS, Tom WL, Lebwohl MG, et al. Efficacy and safety of crisaborole ointment, a novel, nonsteroidal phosphodiesterase 4 (PDE4) inhibitor for the topical treatment of atopic dermatitis (AD) in children and adults. J Am Acad Dermatol 2016;75(3): 494–503.e6.

24. Zane LT, Hughes MH, Shakib S. Tolerability of crisaborole ointment for application on sensitive skin areas: a randomized, double-blind, vehicle-controlled study in healthy volunteers. Am J Clin Dermatol 2016;17(5):519–26.

25. Ghoreschi K, Gadina M. Jakpot! New small molecules in autoimmune and inflammatory diseases. Exp Dermatol 2014;23(1):7–11.

26. Bissonnette R, Papp KA, Poulin Y, et al. Topical tofacitinib for atopic dermatitis: a Phase 2a randomised trial. Br J Dermatol 2016;175(5):902–11.

27. Nakagawa H, Nemoto O, Igarashi A, et al. Efficacy and safety of topical JTE-052, a Janus kinase inhibitor, in Japanese adult patients with moderate-to-severe atopic dermatitis: a phase II, multicentre, randomized, vehicle-controlled clinical study. Br J Dermatol 2018;178(2):424–32.

28. Nakatsuji T, Chen TH, Narala S, et al. Antimicrobials from human skin commensal bacteria protect against Staphylococcus aureus and are deficient in atopic dermatitis. Sci Transl Med 2017;9(378) [pii:eaah4680].

29. Myles IA, Earland NJ, Anderson ED, et al. First-in-human topical microbiome transplantation with Roseomonas mucosa for atopic dermatitis. JCI Insight 2018;3(9) [pii:120608].

30. Kagami S, Saeki H, Komine M, et al. Interleukin-4 and interleukin-13 enhance CCL26 production in a human keratinocyte cell line, HaCaT cells. Clin Exp Immunol 2005;141(3):459–66.

31. Guttman-Yassky E, Dhingra N, Leung DY. New era of biologic therapeutics in atopic dermatitis. Expert Opin Biol Ther 2013;13(4):549–61.

32. Han Y, Chen Y, Liu X, et al. Efficacy and safety of dupilumab for the treatment of adult atopic dermatitis: a meta-analysis of randomized clinical trials. J Allergy Clin Immunol 2017;140(3):888–91.e6.

33. Wang FP, Tang XJ, Wei CQ, et al. Dupilumab treatment in moderate-to-severe atopic dermatitis: a systematic review and meta-analysis. J Dermatol Sci 2018;90(2):190–8.

34. Treister AD, Kraff-Cooper C, Lio PA. Risk factors for dupilumab-associated conjunctivitis in patients with atopic dermatitis. JAMA Dermatol 2018;154(10): 1208–11.

35. Hussein YM, Ahmad AS, Ibrahem MM, et al. Interleukin 13 receptors as biochemical markers in atopic patients. J Investig Allergol Clin Immunol 2011;21(2):101–7.

36. Wollenberg A, Howell MD, Guttman-Yassky E, et al. Treatment of atopic dermatitis with tralokinumab, an anti-IL-13 mAb. J Allergy Clin Immunol 2018. https://doi.org/10.1016/j.jaci.2018.05.029.

37. Ultsch M, Bevers J, Nakamura G, et al. Structural basis of signaling blockade by anti-IL-13 antibody Lebrikizumab. J Mol Biol 2013;425(8):1330–9.

38. Simpson EL, Flohr C, Eichenfield LF, et al. Efficacy and safety of lebrikizumab (an anti-IL-13 monoclonal antibody) in adults with moderate-to-severe atopic dermatitis inadequately controlled by topical corticosteroids: a randomized, placebo-controlled phase II trial (TREBLE). J Am Acad Dermatol 2018;78(5):863–71.e11.

39. Ruzicka T, Hanifin JM, Furue M, et al. Anti-interleukin-31 receptor a antibody for atopic dermatitis. N Engl J Med 2017;376(9):826–35.

40. Szegedi K, Kremer AE, Kezic S, et al. Increased frequencies of IL-31-producing T cells are found in chronic atopic dermatitis skin. Exp Dermatol 2012; 21(6):431–6.

41. Sonkoly E, Muller A, Lauerma AI, et al. IL-31: a new link between T cells and pruritus in atopic skin inflammation. J Allergy Clin Immunol 2006;117(2): 411–7.

42. Liu YJ. Thymic stromal lymphopoietin and OX40 ligand pathway in the initiation of dendritic cell-mediated allergic inflammation. J Allergy Clin Immunol 2007;120(2):238–44 [quiz: 45–6].

43. Nakajima S, Igyarto BZ, Honda T, et al. Langerhans cells are critical in epicutaneous sensitization with protein antigen via thymic stromal lymphopoietin receptor signaling. J Allergy Clin Immunol 2012; 129(4):1048–55.e6.

44. Fujita H, Shemer A, Suarez-Farinas M, et al. Lesional dendritic cells in patients with chronic atopic dermatitis and psoriasis exhibit parallel ability to activate T-cell subsets. J Allergy Clin Immunol 2011;128(3): 574–82.e1-12.

45. Wang YH, Ito T, Wang YH, et al. Maintenance and polarization of human TH2 central memory T cells by thymic stromal lymphopoietin-activated dendritic cells. Immunity 2006;24(6):827–38.

46. Tidwell WJ, Fowler JF Jr. T-cell inhibitors for atopic dermatitis. J Am Acad Dermatol 2018;78(3S1): S67–70.

47. Murakami-Satsutani N, Ito T, Nakanishi T, et al. IL-33 promotes the induction and maintenance of Th2 immune responses by enhancing the function of OX40 ligand. Allergol Int 2014;63(3):443–55.

48. Seltmann J, Roesner LM, von Hesler FW, et al. IL-33 impacts on the skin barrier by downregulating the expression of filaggrin. J Allergy Clin Immunol 2015;135(6):1659–61.e4.

49. Ilves T, Harvima IT. OX40 ligand and OX40 are increased in atopic dermatitis lesions but do not correlate with clinical severity. J Eur Acad Dermatol Venereol 2013;27(2):e197–205.

50. Gauvreau GM, O'Byrne PM, Boulet LP, et al. Effects of an anti-TSLP antibody on allergen-induced asthmatic responses. N Engl J Med 2014;370(22): 2102–10.

51. Guttman-Yassky E, Pavel AB, Estrada Y, et al. 453 GBR 830 induces progressive and sustained changes in atopic dermatitis biomarkers in patient skin lesions. J Invest Dermatol 2018;138(5): S377.

52. Papp KA, Gooderham MJ, Girard G, et al. Phase I randomized study of KHK4083, an anti-OX40 monoclonal antibody, in patients with mild to moderate plaque psoriasis. J Eur Acad Dermatol Venereol 2017;31(8):1324–32.

53. Ogg G. proof-of-concept phase 2a clinical trial of ANB020 (anti-IL-33 antibody) in the treatment of moderate-to-severe atopic dermatitis. AAD annual meeting. San Diego, CA, February 16–8, 2018.

54. Gutowska-Owsiak D, Schaupp AL, Salimi M, et al. IL-17 downregulates filaggrin and affects keratinocyte expression of genes associated with cellular adhesion. Exp Dermatol 2012;21(2):104–10.

55. Howell MD, Kim BE, Gao P, et al. Cytokine modulation of atopic dermatitis filaggrin skin expression. J Allergy Clin Immunol 2007;120(1):150–5.

56. Nograles KE, Zaba LC, Guttman-Yassky E, et al. Th17 cytokines interleukin (IL)-17 and IL-22 modulate distinct inflammatory and keratinocyte-response pathways. Br J Dermatol 2008;159(5): 1092–102.

57. Khattri S, Shemer A, Rozenblit M, et al. Cyclosporine in patients with atopic dermatitis modulates activated inflammatory pathways and reverses epidermal pathology. J Allergy Clin Immunol 2014; 133(6):1626–34.

58. Tintle S, Shemer A, Suarez-Farinas M, et al. Reversal of atopic dermatitis with narrow-band UVB phototherapy and biomarkers for therapeutic response. J Allergy Clin Immunol 2011;128(3):583–93.e1-4.

59. Brunner PM, Khattri S, Garcet S, et al. A mild topical steroid leads to progressive anti-inflammatory effects in the skin of patients with moderate-to-severe atopic dermatitis. J Allergy Clin Immunol 2016;138(1):169–78.

60. Hamilton JD, Suarez-Farinas M, Dhingra N, et al. Dupilumab improves the molecular signature in skin of patients with moderate-to-severe atopic dermatitis. J Allergy Clin Immunol 2014;134(6):1293–300.

61. Khattri S, Brunner PM, Garcet S, et al. Efficacy and safety of ustekinumab treatment in adults with moderate-to-severe atopic dermatitis. Exp Dermatol 2017;26(1):28–35.

62. Guttman-Yassky E, Ungar B, Malik K, et al. Molecular signatures order the potency of topically applied anti-inflammatory drugs in patients with atopic dermatitis. J Allergy Clin Immunol 2017;140(4): 1032–42.e13.

63. Nograles KE, Zaba LC, Shemer A, et al. IL-22-producing "T22" T cells account for upregulated IL-22 in atopic dermatitis despite reduced IL-17-producing TH17 T cells. J Allergy Clin Immunol 2009;123(6):1244–52.e2.

64. Guttman-Yassky E, Brunner PM, Neumann AU, et al. Efficacy and safety of fezakinumab (an IL-22 monoclonal antibody) in adults with moderate-to-severe atopic dermatitis inadequately controlled by conventional treatments: a randomized, double-blind, phase 2a trial. J Am Acad Dermatol 2018;78(5): 872–81.e6.

65. Brunner PM, Pavel AB, Khattri S, et al. Baseline IL22 expression in atopic dermatitis patients stratifies tissue responses to fezakinumab. J Allergy Clin Immunol 2018. https://doi.org/10.1016/j.jaci.2018.07.028.

66. Suarez-Farinas M, Ungar B, Correa da Rosa J, et al. RNA sequencing atopic dermatitis transcriptome profiling provides insights into novel disease mechanisms with potential therapeutic implications. J Allergy Clin Immunol 2015;135(5):1218–27.

67. Suarez-Farinas M, Ungar B, Noda S, et al. Alopecia areata profiling shows TH1, TH2, and IL-23 cytokine activation without parallel TH17/TH22 skewing. J Allergy Clin Immunol 2015;136(5):1277–87.

68. Zheng Y, Danilenko DM, Valdez P, et al. Interleukin-22, a T(H)17 cytokine, mediates IL-23-induced dermal inflammation and acanthosis. Nature 2007; 445(7128):648–51.

69. Papp KA, Langley RG, Lebwohl M, et al. Efficacy and safety of ustekinumab, a human interleukin-12/23 monoclonal antibody, in patients with psoriasis: 52-week results from a randomised, double-blind, placebo-controlled trial (PHOENIX 2). Lancet 2008; 371(9625):1675–84.

70. Shroff A, Guttman-Yassky E. Successful use of ustekinumab therapy in refractory severe atopic dermatitis. JAAD Case Rep 2015;1(1):25–6.

71. Puya R, Alvarez-Lopez M, Velez A, et al. Treatment of severe refractory adult atopic dermatitis with ustekinumab. Int J Dermatol 2012;51(1):115–6.

72. Gu C, Wu L, Li X. IL-17 family: cytokines, receptors and signaling. Cytokine 2013;64(2):477–85.

73. Guttman-Yassky E, Krueger JG. IL-17C: a unique epithelial cytokine with potential for targeting across the spectrum of atopic dermatitis and psoriasis. J Invest Dermatol 2018;138(7):1467–9.

74. Ramirez-Carrozzi V, Sambandam A, Luis E, et al. IL-17C regulates the innate immune function of epithelial cells in an autocrine manner. Nat Immunol 2011; 12(12):1159–66.

75. Hawkes JE, Chan TC, Krueger JG. Psoriasis pathogenesis and the development of novel targeted immune therapies. J Allergy Clin Immunol 2017; 140(3):645–53.

76. Martin DA, Towne JE, Kricorian G, et al. The emerging role of IL-17 in the pathogenesis of psoriasis: preclinical and clinical findings. J Invest Dermatol 2013;133(1):17–26.

77. Thaci D. MOR106, an anti-IL-17C mAb, a potential new approach for treatment of moderate-to-severe atopic dermatitis: phase 1 study. AAD annual meeting. San Diego, USA, 2018.

78. Bao L, Zhang H, Chan LS. The involvement of the JAK-STAT signaling pathway in chronic inflammatory skin disease atopic dermatitis. JAKSTAT 2013;2(3): e24137.

79. Xing L, Dai Z, Jabbari A, et al. Alopecia areata is driven by cytotoxic T lymphocytes and is reversed by JAK inhibition. Nat Med 2014;20(9):1043–9.

80. Guttman-Yassky E, Silverberg JI, Nemoto O, et al. Baricitinib in adult patients with moderate-to-severe atopic dermatitis: a phase 2 parallel, double-blinded, randomized placebo-controlled multiple-dose study. J Am Acad Dermatol 2018. https://doi.org/10.1016/j.jaad.2018.01.018.

81. Guttman-Yassky E. Primary results from a phase 2b, randomized, placebo-controlled trial of upadacitinib for patients with atopic dermatitis. AAD annual meeting. San Diego, USA, 2018.

82. Gooderham M. pf-04965842, a selective jak1 inhibitor, for treatment of moderate-severe atopic dermatitis: a 12 week, randomized, double blind, placebo controlled phase 2 clinical trial. 26th EADV congress. Geneva, Switzerland, September 13–7, 2017.

83. Wollenberg A, Barbarot S, Bieber T, et al. Consensus-based European guidelines for treatment of atopic eczema (atopic dermatitis) in adults and children: part II. J Eur Acad Dermatol Venereol 2018;32(6):850–78.

84. Glatzer F, Gschwandtner M, Ehling S, et al. Histamine induces proliferation in keratinocytes from patients with atopic dermatitis through the histamine 4 receptor. J Allergy Clin Immunol 2013;132(6): 1358–67.

85. De Benedetto A, Yoshida T, Fridy S, et al. Histamine and skin barrier: are histamine antagonists useful for the prevention or treatment of atopic dermatitis? J Clin Med 2015;4(4):741–55.

Treatment Update of Autoimmune Blistering Diseases

Khalaf Kridin, MD, PhD[a], Christine Ahn, MD[b],
William C. Huang, MD, MPH[b], Ahmed Ansari, BS[c],
Naveed Sami, MD[d],*

KEYWORDS

- Autoimmune blistering diseases • Rituximab • Treatment • Emerging

KEY POINTS

- Rituximab has become a conventional treatment of pemphigus with an FDA labeled indication in 2018.
- Anecdotal data indicate that Rituximab is also a promising treatment of autoimmune subepidermal blistering diseases.
- Rituximab can be used as a rescue treatment in recalcitrant autoimmune blistering diseases in children.
- Progress continues to be made in refining standardized disease severity scores for autoimmune blistering diseases.
- Numerous new emerging treatments hold promise with biologics and other targeted immunotherapies.

INTRODUCTION

The aim of the treatment in autoimmune blistering diseases (AIBDs) is to induce and maintain remission, which clinically corresponds to the cessation of new vesicle formation, healing of old erosions, and completion of tapering of treatment.[1,2] Subsequently, a substantial challenge is to prevent relapse in the long term and avoid adverse events associated with the prolonged use of corticosteroids and immunosuppressive agents.[3] Given the rarity of this group of diseases, progress in randomized controlled trials (RCTs) has been slow. Rituximab emerged as a promising therapeutic agent, and has recently led to its US Food and Drug Administration (FDA) indication for the treatment of pemphigus. Rituximab has been reported to a lesser extent in subepidermal autoimmune blistering diseases (s-AIBDs).[4,5] In addition, several promising novel therapeutic agents have been recently evolving for the treatment of pemphigus and other s-AIBDs.[6]

This article aims to present an updated review of the literature on the role of rituximab in the treatment of AIBDs, as well as on the emerging therapies for this group of potentially life-threatening tissue-specific autoimmune diseases.

Disclosure: The authors have nothing to disclose.
[a] Department of Dermatology, Rambam Health Care Campus, POB 9602, Haifa 31096, Israel; [b] Department of Dermatology, Wake Forest School of Medicine, Wake Forest University, 4618 Country Club Road, Winston-Salem, NC 27104, USA; [c] College of Medicine (Lake Nona), University of Central Florida, 6850 Lake Nona Boulevard, Orlando, FL 32827, USA; [d] Department of Medicine, University of Central Florida, Health Sciences Campus at Lake Nona, 2627 Northampton Avenue, Orlando, FL 32827-7408, USA
* Corresponding author. Department of Dermatology, UCF Health-3rd Floor, 9975 Tavistock Boulevard, Orlando, FL 32828, USA
E-mail addresses: naveed.sami@ucf.edu; nsderm@gmail.com

Dermatol Clin 37 (2019) 215–228
https://doi.org/10.1016/j.det.2018.12.003
0733-8635/19/© 2018 Elsevier Inc. All rights reserved.

RITUXIMAB UPDATE
Rituximab in Pemphigus Vulgaris

Efficacy and safety

The first report of the successful use of rituximab for the treatment of pemphigus vulgaris (PV) was in 2002. Salopek and colleagues[7] reported a case of recalcitrant, life-threatening PV with nearly 100% body surface area (BSA) involvement failing to respond to multidrug immunosuppressive therapy.[7] The mechanism through which rituximab affects PV is 2-fold: B-cell progenitors of autoantibody-secreting plasma cells are depleted and desmoglein (Dsg)-specific CD4$^+$ T cells are downregulated.[8]

Since this initial report, the clinical use of rituximab has become part of more conventional treatment as both a rescue and first-line treatment in the treatment algorithm of pemphigus. Based on its clinical use in other diseases, 2 different dosing protocols for rituximab have been established. The conventional dosing of a single cycle of rituximab for the treatment of lymphoma consists of 4 infusions of rituximab at 375 mg/m^2 each given 1 week apart. By contrast, the conventional dosing of a single cycle for rheumatoid arthritis (RA) consists of 1 g for 2 infusions given 2 weeks apart.[9]

In a recent meta-analysis evaluating the efficacy of rituximab for pemphigus after one cycle, disease control and remission on adjuvant treatment was observed within 1 month and 6 months respectively, with an overall 76% of patients achieving complete remission. The mean duration of remission was reported to be about 15 months with 40% of patients having a relapse.[9] Although there are no published studies that have compared rituximab with a combination of systemic corticosteroids and conventional oral treatments in the same study, overall similar rates of remission have been observed.[10] Results of a recently completed study comparing rituximab with mycophenolate mofetil in severe PV are pending.

Dosing

There is no clear consensus on the dosing schedules of rituximab in PV. The lymphoma and RA protocols have been described as high-dose protocols. The RA protocol (fixed-dose) has been slightly favored over the lymphoma protocol. Authors provide rationale for this approach based on the different biological behavior of B cells in lymphoma compared with autoimmune diseases such as RA and PV.[11] In addition, a pharmacokinetic study of rituximab in RA patients demonstrated no benefit for BSA-dependent dosing of rituximab.[12] Studies have also reported the use of a combination or modified version of these dosing protocols, and have investigated the use of a low-dose RA protocol of 500 mg for 2 infusions given 2 weeks apart or only 2 infusions with the lymphoma protocol.

The rate of clinical response was comparable between the RA and lymphoma protocol treatment groups. Though not statistically significant, a shorter time to disease control and remission along with higher clinical remission was observed with the lymphoma protocol. Patients in the RA protocol group had a higher rate of relapse (65% compared with 41% in the lymphoma protocol group) in a similar time period (16–17 months), and 80% received additional infusions in the RA group (compared with 24% of patients in the lymphoma protocol group).[13]

Studies have also reported the use of a combination or modified version of these dosing protocols, using a lower-dose regimen of the RA protocol of 500 mg for 2 infusions given 2 weeks apart or only 2 infusions with the lymphoma protocol. When higher-dose and lower-dose RA protocols were compared, the clinical remission rate was comparable, and adverse events associated with 500-mg dosing were lower than with 1-g dosing.[13] However, certain outcome measures seem to favor the higher-dose protocols, with a shorter time to clinical remission in addition to lower relapse rate and more sustained response when compared with lower-dose protocols.

In addition to a standardized dosing protocol, the optimal duration of treatment has not been established for PV. Despite demonstrating clinical outcomes similar to those for the lymphoma protocol, the RA protocol is limited by the high rate of rebound when treated with only one cycle (2 infusions). In a retrospective study of patients receiving lymphoma protocol dosing (375 mg/m^2) for variable total infusions, complete remission rates were higher (73%) and relapse rates lower (0%) in patients receiving 3 or more infusions, compared with patients receiving 2 or fewer infusions (relapse rate 67%).[14] Heelan and colleagues[15] demonstrated the long-term efficacy and tolerability of a modified RA protocol for rituximab in patients with PV and pemphigus foliaceus (PF). In their study, 64 patients were treated with 1 g for 2 infusions spaced 2 weeks apart, followed by a single dose of 1 g or 500 mg 6 months or more after induction if clinically indicated. Complete response was observed in 70% of patients.[15] Additional rituximab infusions for prophylactic measures to prevent relapses in clinically clear patients does not appear to have any benefit in preventing later relapses.[16]

Treatment paradigm

Based on increasing evidence of the clinical benefits of rituximab, there has been a shift in the current treatment paradigm for PV. First-line therapy for PV usually involves oral corticosteroids and adjuvant immunosuppressive agents such as mycophenolate mofetil or azathioprine. Second-line or third-line or "rescue" treatment options include plasmapheresis/immunoadsorption (IA), intravenous cyclophosphamide, intravenous immunoglobulin (IVIg), and rituximab. In the therapeutic ladder established by Strowd and colleagues,[17] the authors suggest first-line therapy consisting of high-dose oral corticosteroids with the early addition of adjuvant steroid-sparing agents such as mycophenolate mofetil. However, some studies have demonstrated that patients treated with adjuvant therapy before treatment with rituximab have higher rates of relapse.[15] In a retrospective study of 150 patients with pemphigus treated with a single cycle of rituximab, increased duration of disease before receiving treatment was associated with failure to achieve complete remission.[18] Other factors, including rapid taper or discontinuation of prerituximab conventional therapy, may also contribute to a relapse. A recent study demonstrated that continuation of lower dosages of before rituximab conventional treatment after achieving clinical control with rituximab may help reduce the risk of relapse in pemphigus patients.[19]

Numerous reports describe the use of rituximab as a first-line single agent. These cases describe good clinical outcomes and high rates of remission, but also require longer dosing regimens as frequently as weekly for 8 weeks and monthly for 4 months.[20] In a multicenter RCT, patients with newly diagnosed pemphigus were treated with either prednisone (1.0 or 1.5 mg/kg/d) tapered over 12 to 18 months or rituximab (RA protocol followed by 500 mg at months 12 and 18) and oral prednisone (0.5 or 1.0 mg/kg/d) tapered over 3 to 6 months. Eighty-nine percent of patients treated with rituximab and short-term prednisone were in complete remission off therapy at 24 months, compared with 34% of patients treated with prednisone alone.[4] Further studies corroborate the safety and efficacy of rituximab and oral corticosteroid therapy as first-line therapy for patients with pemphigus. Cho and colleagues[21] describe 9 moderate-to-severe pemphigus patients initiated on systemic corticosteroids (1.0 mg/kg/d) followed by 500 mg of rituximab for 4 weekly infusions, with tapering of corticosteroids by 6 months. Relapse occurred in 8 of 9 patients, however, and patients received additional rituximab monotherapy, azathioprine monotherapy, or rituximab and corticosteroid combination therapy.[21]

Rituximab has also been suggested as a potential first-line therapy for patients in whom systemic corticosteroids are contraindicated. In one study, 5 patients were treated with rituximab fixed-dose regimen (4 patients) and weight-based lymphoma protocol dosing (1 patient) and daily applications of topical clobetasol. Patients achieved complete or near complete healing of disease at a mean of 15 weeks after the first infusion. This small series shows potential for rituximab as a first-line therapy when oral corticosteroids are contraindicated.[22] In summary, the current reported literature may suggest that the early use of higher doses of rituximab may favor better long-term clinical outcomes in the treatment of adult pemphigus patients.

Rituximab in the Treatment of Subepidermal Autoimmune Blistering Diseases

Rituximab has been used in multiple s-AIBDs including mucous membrane pemphigoid (MMP), bullous pemphigoid (BP), epidermolysis bullosa acquisita (EBA), pemphigoid gestationis (PG), and dermatitis herpetiformis (DH).[23–39] Although the experience in these diseases is not as extensively reported as for pemphigus, most patients have been treated with both the lymphoma and RA protocol with a handful being treated with low-dose rituximab infusions.

The largest reported cohort of s-AIBDs treated with rituximab has been in MMP, which can have variations of multiple mucosal involvement and, hence, possibly a heterogeneous disease. The number of patients treated with the lymphoma RA protocols has been comparable with a greater than 90% clinical response, with the vast majority in clinical remission at some stage during the treatment process. The time to disease control has ranged between 3 and 10 months.[23,24] However, relapse rates have been relatively high, ranging between 42% and 100% in different studies.[24,25] The difference in delay in relapse can possibly be attributed to adjuvant oral conventional treatment being continued with rituximab.[24]

BP primarily presents in the elderly population. Hence, rituximab has been used with caution because of the potential higher risk of intolerability and certain adverse reactions. The first report of rituximab in an adult patient with BP was in 2007 with the lymphoma protocol.[26] Since then, the RA protocol has been more widely used in the treatment of refractory BP as rescue therapy. Ninety percent of patients have achieved clinical remission (complete remission [CR] or partial remission [PR]) with either protocol. Relapse rates have varied widely between 12% and 60% with no protocol predilection.[5,27–33] A study by Cho and colleagues[34] evaluated the utility of rituximab as first-line therapy in comparison with prednisolone as monotherapy. Patients in the rituximab group received 4 weekly infusions of rituximab 500 mg and prednisolone 0.5 mg/kg daily (tapered following disease control). The control group received a similar starting dose of prednisone for 6 months. Twelve of 13 patients in the rituximab group achieved CR, whereas 10 of 19 patients in the prednisone-only group achieved CR. Moreover, 8 patients in the rituximab group maintained CR off therapy with 4 of these having sustained maintenance during the follow-up period of more than 2 years. The other 4 patients had mild relapses. Adverse reactions including infection rates were less frequently observed in the rituximab group (4 of 13 patients) compared with the prednisone-only group (10 of 19 patients) along with a lower 1-year mortality in the rituximab group (2 of 13) than in the prednisone group (7 of 19). This study offered encouraging support for the use of combination therapy with rituximab as first-line therapy.[34]

EBA is a less common AIBD that can be more refractory to therapy. There have been a total of 19 reported EBA patients treated with rituximab, with the overwhelming majority receiving the RA protocol as the only rescue agent. Only one patient has achieved CR, whereas 80% have shown improvement with a clinical response.[35]

PG, a rare AIBD most commonly affecting women in the sixth to ninth month of gestation and early postpartum period, usually spontaneously resolves after delivery, but may persist in the postpartum period. Cianchini and colleagues[36] reported a case of a 31-year-old woman with recalcitrant PG, which persisted after delivery and failed to respond to high-dose systemic prednisone, azathioprine, and dapsone. The patient had CR with a modified lymphoma protocol without any adverse effects. In addition, Tourte and colleagues[37] reported the use of rituximab as "prophylactic therapy" in a 36-year-old woman during the beginning of her fifth pregnancy. She had developed PG in 2 previous pregnancies resulting in complications and, hence, subsequently received the RA protocol in week 9 and week 11 of her fifth pregnancy. It is difficult to state whether rituximab definitely prevented her PG relapse and subsequent potential complications. However, a significant decline in anti-BP180 autoantibody titers was observed.[37] Although no complications were observed in both PG cases, it is still recommended to avoid rituximab during pregnancy, and cautious usage may be exercised if needed for severe, recurrent disease. Further studies are needed to define its dosing and safety profile.

DH generally responds well to a gluten-free diet and dapsone. However, for refractory cases treatment options are limited. A recent report described the use of rituximab (lymphoma protocol) in an elderly refractory DH patient. CR was maintained at his 18-month follow-up normalization of antitissue transglutaminase autoantibodies.[38]

Low-dose rituximab has been used primarily in MMP and BP, with a higher CR rate. However, it is difficult to make any definitive conclusion because this has been reported in only a handful of cases. Reports of adverse events in the use of rituximab in s-AIBDs have been few. The most common side effect has been infection in MMP, BP, and EBA.[23,26,35,39]

Rituximab in Pediatric Patients

Pediatric pemphigus and pemphigoid are rare, and can be particularly challenging to treat in children because of the significant morbidity associated with treatment. The experience with rituximab in refractory AIBDs in children is limited.[26,40–46] The first reports of rituximab to treat pediatric patients with an autoimmune bullous disease was in children with BP.[40,44] All but one of the children with BP, whose ages ranged from 5 months to 10 years, responded to the lymphoma protocol. One child developed drug-induced fever after the initial infusion and was subsequently treated with a lower dose (187 mg/m[2]).[40] Although the reported experience with rituximab in pemphigus in children is not as extensive as in adults, the response and tolerance to rituximab has been favorable, with remission being achieved after 4 to 7 months.[41] Rituximab treatment protocols have varied, with patients receiving between 2 and 7 infusions of 375 mg/m[2] or 2 fixed doses of 500 mg administered 2 weeks apart.[41,42] Response and relapse rates in pediatric pemphigus and BP have been comparable. However, it is difficult to conclude whether lower-dose protocols can potentially result in a higher risk of earlier relapse. Whereas hypersensitivity reactions have been the most common adverse effect, infections have been less frequently reported in children with AIBDs treated with rituximab.[26] Few children have received postrituximab monthly IVIg as a short-term and long-term maintenance treatment because of hypogammaglobulinemia and decreased immunization antibody titers, respectively.[26,43] For severe recalcitrant disease, rituximab may be a therapeutic option with good efficacy and a safer side-effect profile in children.[44–46] However, further studies are needed to evaluate exact dosing (higher versus lower) and rituximab's role as a first-line or rescue treatment in children with AIBDs.

Combination Treatments

Severe recalcitrant autoimmune bullous diseases have been treated with combination therapy. IVIg and plasmapheresis were initially combined in treating PV and BP.[47,48] Subsequent publications have reported the experience using a combination of immunoadsorption and IVIg with rituximab in pemphigus and s-AIBDs.[49–61] A combination of IA or IVIg with rituximab can help, in both arresting acute progression of disease and preventing a rebound exacerbation.

Rituximab in combination with IA has been used in the treatment of pemphigus, BP, MMP, and EBA. Both lymphoma and RA protocols were used with IA. However, the number of IA treatments received by patients has varied between studies. The vast majority of patients treated with IA and rituximab were those with severe progressive pemphigus, with a positive initial response observed as early as within 1 month of initiating the combination treatments.[49–51] Although far fewer patients with s-AIBDs have been treated with this combination, a favorable but slower response was reported. CR was generally observed after 6 months.[52,53] The most common reported side effect was severe infection.[53]

Combination of rituximab and IVIg (2 g/cycle) has been reported with unique protocols. The rituximab dosing in these studies has been primarily based on BSA involvement, with most patients receiving 10 to 12 infusions over a 6-month period. Although a clinical response was reported in all treated patients with pemphigus, approximately one-third of the patients relapsed.[54–57] Fewer relapses were reported in patients with BP, MMP, and EBA who were treated with this combination. However, these patients also were treated long-term with more IVIg infusions.[58–61] One study reported progression of ocular cicatricial pemphigoid in 50% of their treated patients with the RA protocol and fewer IVIg infusions.[61] The cost of treatment would be significantly high if these modalities were combined. Hence, this combination may best be used in patients with severe progressive AIBDs who have not responded to rituximab as a first-line or second-line agent in combination with other conventional adjuvants.

Severity Score Measurements

Outcome measures are an important part of clinical assessment, both for individual patient care and for large multicenter studies. Several tools have been established to measure disease activity, severity, and impact on quality of life in AIBD patients. The pemphigus disease area index (PDAI), autoimmune bullous skin disorder intensity score (ABSIS), and PV activity score (PVAS) have been used to measure disease activity.[62] The use of validated clinical severity tools that have high interrater reliability and correlate with objective measures such as antibody titers is important for conducting large-scale multicenter studies. In one cross-sectional study, these 3 tools were assessed for interrater reliability and correlated with autoantibody titers. The highest interrater reliability was observed with the PDAI, followed by the ABSIS and PVAS.[63] The PDAI and ABSIS can also be used to categorize pemphigus into moderate, significant, and extensive subtypes.[62] Recently, a separate score to assess the severity of oral disease called the oral disease severity score (ODSS) was validated in a study of 15 patients with oral PV.[64] Compared with other tools such as the PDAI, ABSIS, and PGA (physician's global assessment), the ODSS appears to have higher interrater and intrarater reliability, and is thus helpful in further characterizing oral disease activity.[64] The ABQOL (autoimmune bullous disease quality of life) is a validated tool that quantifies the burden of autoimmune bullous diseases and its treatments on patients' quality of life.[65]

EMERGING TREATMENTS BEYOND RITUXIMAB
Pemphigus

Next-generation anti-CD20 monoclonal antibodies

New generations of anti-CD20 monoclonal antibodies that are either humanized or fully human have been developed in recent years to circumvent the immunogenicity associated with rituximab. The degree of associated immunogenicity was alleged to embody a decisive role in determining the efficacy and tolerability of the treatment.[66] Other rationales motivating the production of these agents are to alleviate the adverse events observed with rituximab exposure and to reduce its costs by using subcutaneous routes of administration. The humanized forms include ocrelizumab, veltuzumab, and obinutuzumab, whereas ofatumumab is currently the only available fully human anti-CD20 monoclonal antibody.[66] These agents are also categorized as type I (rituximab, ocrelizumab, veltuzumab, and ofatumumab) or type II (obinutuzumab and tositumomab) in accordance with the cellular response on binding. Whereas type I antibodies induce clustering of CD20 and recruitment and activation of complement system leading to a substantial complement-dependent cytotoxic (CDC) response, type II antibodies mainly induce direct cell death with a marginal CDC response.

Only veltuzumab and ofatumumab were linked to the treatment of patients with pemphigus.[67,68]

Veltuzumab Veltuzumab is a type I, second-generation humanized, anti-CD20 monoclonal antibody characterized by a greater binding avidity and larger effect on CDC when compared with rituximab.[66] A major advantage of veltuzumab over rituximab is its ability to be administered subcutaneously in low doses.[69] Subcutaneous veltuzumab (two 320-mg doses 2 weeks apart) was administered on a compassionate-use basis in one patient with PV refractory to rituximab. The patient experienced CR off therapy at 22 months but relapsed at 24 months. A second cycle of veltuzumab at the same dosing regimen led to remission persisting for 9 months later until the end of the follow-up. Veltuzumab was granted orphan status designation for pemphigus in 2015.[70]

Ofatumumab Ofatumumab is a type I, fully human, anti-CD20 monoclonal antibody binding to an epitope distinct from that recognized by rituximab, and is characterized by greater CDC response and apoptosis induction when compared with rituximab.[71] A phase III randomized placebo-controlled trial of subcutaneous ofatumumab recruiting 35 patients with moderate or severe pemphigus was recently terminated after this agent was acquired by a different sponsor (NCT01920477).[66]

B-cell activating factor and a proliferation-inducing ligand inhibitors
B-cell activating factor (BAFF) is a member of the tumor necrosis factor (TNF) superfamily cytokine and is an important activator of B-cell differentiation.[72] A proliferation-inducing ligand (APRIL), another TNF superfamily ligand, is also implicated in B-cell ontogeny.[73] BAFF and APRIL were demonstrated to contribute to the switching of immunoglobulin to the IgG, IgE, and IgA subclasses.[74,75] Unlike the important correlation between BAFF levels and the activity of some autoimmune diseases, namely RA and systemic lupus erythematosus,[76] serum levels of BAFF and APRIL were not elevated in patients with PV.[77] In addition, rituximab use in PV patients resulted in a significant elevation of serum BAFF levels but a decrease in anti-Dsg1 and anti-Dsg3 autoantibody titers.[78] In the same study, an inverse association between BAFF levels and peripheral CD19+ levels in PV patients treated with rituximab was found. Although BAFF and APRIL were not established as dominant players in the immunopathogenesis of PV, further studies are warranted to clarify their role in this disease. Clearly an improved mechanistic understanding of the role of BAFF in PV pathogenesis is necessary before inhibitors of this factor, such as belimumab, can be considered for the treatment of PV.[79]

Chimeric antigen receptor therapy
Dsg-specific immune suppression by specifically targeting B and T cells involved in the production of pathogenic pemphigus autoantibodies has recently been claiming a substantial place in therapeutic strategies. The possibility of using modified chimeric antigen receptor therapy to target Dsg3-specific B cells was recently proposed; human T cells were engineered to express a chimeric autoantibody receptor (CAAR) consisting of Dsg3. In murine model, Dsg3 CAAR-T cells exhibit specific cytotoxicity against B cells bearing anti-Dsg3 B-cell receptors in vitro and specifically target Dsg3-specific B cells in vivo. This strategy is supposed to deplete anti-Dsg3 memory B cells, directly and indirectly, and deplete Dsg3-specific short-lived plasma cells that produce the pathogenic autoantibodies. CAAR-T cells may provide a valuable approach to specifically target autoreactive B cells in PV without causing general immunosuppression.[80] Given that the target antigens and pathophysiologic mechanisms of pemphigus have been well characterized, this innovative approach would signify a revolutionary therapeutic strategy.

T-cell immunotherapy
T-cell activation is necessary for the initiation and coordination of the autoantibody response in pemphigus.[81,82] It is plausible to hinder with T-cell function at several points by using monoclonal antibodies to block specific accessory coreceptors, cytokines, or costimulatory molecules.

Antigen-specific T cells and B cells must interact via the molecules CD154 and CD40, respectively, to produce autoantibodies. Blocking CD154 by the use of an anti-CD154 monoclonal antibody in a mouse model prevented the production of anti-Dsg3 IgG and the subsequent development of the PV phenotype.[83] In other mouse models, the transfer of Dsg3-specific CD4+ T cells can result in a PV phenotype, with interleukin-4 upregulation playing a substantial role in this process.[84]

Altered peptide ligands (APLs) may be used in an immune-based treatment strategy targeting the T-cell level. APLs are peptide analogs with one or more amino acid substitutions at major T-cell receptor contact residues. APLs could be engineered to prevent the interaction between autoreactive T cells and autoantigen peptides presenting on disease-associated HLA class II molecules, and consequently inhibit the start of the autoimmune process. Instead, APLs could induce an incomplete response by antigen-specific T cells, causing T-cell functional tolerance. A phase I clinical trial in PV patients studied the effects of systemic PI-0824, a Dsg3 peptide found to be immunodominant in a small subset of patients. The aim of this therapeutic strategy is to induce T-cell tolerance and abrogate the source of T-cell help required for the production of autoantibodies directed against Dsg3. Neither a significant decline in anti-Dsg3 antibodies nor a phenotypical outcome was observed in this study following the intravenous administration of Dsg3 peptides.[85]

P38MAPK signaling pathway inhibitor
IgG-induced phosphorylation was found to activate p38 mitogen-activated protein kinase (p38MAPK) and heat-shock protein (HSP) 27, which causes downstream remodeling of the actin cytoskeleton and retraction of keratin and contributes to the impairment in cell-cell adhesion. This signaling pathway is initiated following IgG autoantibody binding to keratinocytes and may lead to acantholysis.[86] Experiments using human cultured keratinocytes had suggested that inhibition of p38MAPK prevents the phosphorylation of HSP27, and therefore averts early cytoskeletal changes.[86] This hypothesis was substantiated when SB202190, an inhibitor of p38MAPK, was found to avert blister formation by inhibiting IgG-activated signaling in a mouse model of PV.[87] Enhancement of anti-Dsg1 IgG antibodies and blister formation in PF in a p38MAPK-dependent mechanism also emphasizes the role of p38MAP in the pathomechanism of pemphigus.[88] However, although p38MAPK signaling pathway inhibition protects against blistering in PV, Mao and colleagues[89] demonstrated that blistering could also occur in mice lacking the major p38MAPK isoform. This may lead to the conclusion that p38MAPK is not essential for the loss of intercellular adhesion in PV, but may function downstream to enhance blistering.

Studies examining p38MAPK inhibitors in animal models reported severe adverse effects (mainly hepatotoxicity, undefined gastrointestinal toxicity, and unusual inflammatory response in the central nervous system).[90] To date there has only been one clinical trial performed to assess the use of oral p38MAPK inhibitors in PV patients. The trial was terminated early (because of high hepatotoxicity) without providing meaningful conclusions regarding the efficacy of this agent.[79]

Bruton's tyrosine kinase inhibitor
Bruton's tyrosine kinase (BTK) inhibition targets several pathways and cell types implicated in inflammation and autoimmunity. These include modulation of B-cell receptor-mediated B-cell pathways, as well as inhibition of FcR-induced cytokine release from monocytes and macrophages, FcεR-induced mast cell degranulation, and granulocyte migration.[91] Mutations in the gene encoding BTK result in X-linked agammaglobulinemia type 1, an immunodeficiency associated with failure to produce mature B lymphocytes, and is associated with a failure in immunoglobulin heavy chain rearrangement.[92]

Initial results of a phase II open-label cohort study examining the reversible covalent BTK inhibitor PRN1008 in adult patients with PV disclosed promising efficacy and steroid-sparing effect.[93] The reversible, covalent, oral, small-molecule BTK inhibitor, PRN473, demonstrated a good response in canine PF.[91] In 2017, PRN1008 was granted orphan drug designation by the FDA for the treatment of PV patients.

FAS ligand inhibitor
A recent experimental study demonstrated that soluble Fas ligand plays a critical role in the pathomechanisms leading to blister formation in pemphigus.[94] Fas ligand is significantly upregulated and released from keratinocytes following the binding of pathogenic autoantibodies and contributes to the activation of caspases leading to acantholysis. Of interest, animal models lacking soluble Fas ligand do not experience autoantibody-induced acantholysis.[94] Recently, an Italian group developed a novel antisoluble Fas ligand human monoclonal antibody (PC111) for the treatment of pemphigus. This antibody is characterized by a very low potential of immunogenicity, favorable chemical and physical stability, and high binding affinity. In 2012, PC111 gained the orphan drug designation for the treatment of pemphigus by the European Medicine Agency. The compound is currently being investigated in in vivo preclinical studies.

Neonatal Fc receptor inhibitors
Experimental evidence suggests that neonatal FC receptor (FcRn) plays a notable role in several immunologic mechanisms such as antigen-antibody complex clearance, major histocompatibility complex (MHC) class II antigen presentation, and MHC class I dendritic cell function.[95] Li and colleagues[96] have postulated that the therapeutic efficacy of IVIg in animal models of pemphigus is mediated via FcRn. The aforementioned studies had suggested FcRn as a promising therapeutic target for treating this IgG-mediated autoimmune disease by the prevention of persistent autoantigen presentation and consequently the inhibition

of long-term autoantibody production, as well as by enhancing the catabolism of pathogenic auto-antibodies. SYNT001, An IgG4 monoclonal antibody blocking the binding site of human FcRn, has been recently developed.

A phase 1B multicenter open-label study is currently ongoing to evaluate the efficacy of SYNT001 in the treatment of patients with pemphigus. Preliminary findings in 3 participants demonstrated that the agent is associated with high tolerability, a decrease in circulating anti-Dsg titers, and a good clinical response. These promising findings led the FDA to grant an orphan drug designation to SYNT001 for the treatment of pemphigus in September 2018.

Bullous Pemphigoid

Omalizumab
Omalizumab is a humanized IgG monoclonal antibody that targets the receptor-binding site on circulating IgE, and therefore reduces the binding of IgE to its high-affinity receptors (FcεRI receptors) on mast cells, basophils, and other inflammatory cells.[97] It additionally decreases the expression of FcεRI on immune effector cells.[98] These mechanisms of action reduce the release of inflammatory mediators from these cells and alleviate the inflammatory response. In dermatology, omalizumab has been used in the treatment of IgE-mediated conditions such as chronic urticaria and severe atopic dermatitis.[68,99] Given the accumulating evidence that suggests an important role of anti-BP180 IgE autoantibodies in the pathogenesis of BP,[100,101] omalizumab emerged as a promising therapeutic option in BP. Reasonable efficacy and safety of omalizumab was reported in case reports and one case series of patients with BP.[102–109] In a case series of 6 patients with BP, a therapeutic benefit was observed in 5 patients, of whom 3 responded to omalizumab as monotherapy and 2 as a steroid-sparing agent.[102] None of these patients had adverse reactions to the drug.[102] A pilot, phase IV, open-label randomized trial is currently ongoing to compare the efficacy of treatment with omalizumab with the standard treatment with systemic corticosteroids.[110]

Bertilimumab
Bertilimumab is a human monoclonal antibody targeting eotaxin-1, a potent chemoattractant of eosinophils and important regulator of eosinophil overall function.[111] Eotaxin-1 was found to be upregulated in the serum and blister fluid of BP patient.[112] In light of the substantial role that eosinophils may play in the etiopathogenesis of BP,[113,114] targeting eotaxin-1 may be a beneficial therapeutic approach.

A pilot, phase II, open-label, single-group trial aiming to assess the efficacy and safety of bertilimumab in BP is currently ongoing, and its preliminary results are satisfactory. Recently, the FDA has designated bertilimumab as an orphan drug for the treatment of BP.

Dimethyl fumarate
Dimethyl fumarate (DMF) is an oral immunomodulatory agent approved for the treatment of moderate-to-severe plaque psoriasis and multiple sclerosis, and characterized by a favorable safety profile.[115] DMF may exert its therapeutic effect possibly by activating a nuclear factor erythroid 2-related factor 2 (NRF2) that regulates certain "antioxidant" genes involved in protecting cells from damage, as well as by inhibiting the infiltration of neutrophils and monocytes into the skin.[116–118] A recent study demonstrated that DMF is effective in a preclinical model of BP-like EBA.[119] A randomized, double-blind, placebo-controlled trial aiming to evaluate the safety and the efficacy of DMF as adjuvant therapy in BP has been launched recently and is expected to recruit 120 patients. In 2016, an orphan designation was granted by the European Commission for DMF in the treatment of BP.

C5a-LTB4 axis inhibition
Recent experimental studies have demonstrated that C5a is a strong chemoattractant for granulocytes and exerts an important role in the initiation of tissue inflammation in response to the deposition of IgG autoantibodies. Correspondingly, mice deficient in its precursor C5 or its receptor C5aR1 do not experience granulocyte recruitment and tissue inflammation.[120] In mouse models of pemphigoid, the recruitment of neutrophils into the skin was hindered significantly even when only one of the mediators of the C5a-LTB4 axis or their receptors were lacking, which prevented the expression of the clinical phenotype of the disease.[121] These findings signify that this axis may embody a highly attractive therapeutic target in the treatment of pemphigoid diseases. Novel drugs inhibiting one or both of the aforementioned mediators are expected to be licensed in the near future.

Epidermolysis Bullosa Acquisita

Heat-shock protein 90 inhibitors
HSPs are chaperones with an important role in maintaining the physiologic cellular functions by averting misfolding and aggregation of nascent proteins. Inhibition of the cell stress-inducible

chaperone HSP90 has recently emerged as a promising therapeutic option in cancer and autoimmunity.[122,123] Several observations lend weight to the use of this strategy in EBA: (1) the therapeutic efficacy of HSP90 inhibitors in preclinical EBA mouse models, reflected in the induction of clinical recovery associated with suppressed autoantibody production[124]; (2) the immunosuppressive effects on B and T lymphocytes, which are involved centrally in the pathogenesis of EBA[123–125]; and (3) the increased expression of HSP90 in the skin of patients with pemphigoid diseases.[125,126]

This therapeutic approach has been recently used in mouse models of chronic inflammatory diseases such as systemic lupus erythematosus[127] and arthritis.[128] Anti-HSP90 treatment is currently being tested in clinical trials for the treatment of patients with cancer because of its inhibitory effects on malignant cells. However, clinical trials using these compounds in the treatment of EBA have yet to be launched.

Phosphatidylinositol-3-kinase δ inhibitor

The phosphatidylinositol-3-kinase (PI3K) pathway is activated in several inflammatory and cancerous conditions, and the effectiveness of pharmacologic inhibition or genetic inactivation of this pathway has been evidenced in several preclinical models of inflammatory and malignant conditions.[129] PI3Kδ has been found to be implicated in B-cell and neutrophil cellular functions. Because both cell types contribute to the pathomechanism of EBA, targeting PI3Kδ may be of assistance in treating the disease. A recent study examined the efficacy of LAS191954, an oral selective PI3Kδ inhibitor, in an experimental EBA mouse model.[130] This study revealed that chronic administration of this compound improves the clinical phenotype in a dose-dependent manner, with a significant superiority over high-dose corticosteroid.[130]

Other targets

Targeting the C5a-LTB4 axis, DMF, and the P38MAPK signaling pathway was proposed as a putative therapeutic approach for EBA. These three strategies were discussed thoroughly with respect to BP and pemphigus, respectively.

SUMMARY

There have been significant advances in the treatment of AIBD, and experts see great promise in rituximab with regard to good clinical outcomes and safety profile. In addition, molecules directed against several immunologic pathways have offered possibilities for future implementation in new therapies for these tissue-specific autoimmune diseases.

REFERENCES

1. Murrell DF, Dick S, Ahmed AR, et al. Consensus statement on definitions of disease, end points, and therapeutic response for pemphigus. J Am Acad Dermatol 2008;58(6):1043–6.
2. Feliciani C, Joly P, Jonkman MF, et al. Management of bullous pemphigoid: the European Dermatology Forum consensus in collaboration with the European Academy of Dermatology and Venereology. Br J Dermatol 2015. https://doi.org/10.1111/bjd.13717.
3. Hertl M, Jedlickova H, Karpati S, et al. Pemphigus. S2 Guideline for diagnosis and treatment - guided by the European Dermatology Forum (EDF) in cooperation with the European Academy of Dermatology and Venereology (EADV). J Eur Acad Dermatol Venereol 2015;29(3):405–14.
4. Joly P, Maho-Vaillant M, Prost-Squarcioni C, et al. First-line rituximab combined with short-term prednisone versus prednisone alone for the treatment of pemphigus (Ritux 3): a prospective, multicentre, parallel-group, open-label randomised trial. Lancet 2017;389(10083):2031–40.
5. Lamberts A, Euverman HI, Terra JB, et al. Effectiveness and safety of rituximab in recalcitrant pemphigoid diseases. Front Immunol 2018;9. https://doi.org/10.3389/fimmu.2018.00248.
6. Kridin K. Emerging treatment options for the management of pemphigus vulgaris. Ther Clin Risk Manag 2018;14:757–78.
7. Salopek TG, Logsetty S, Tredget EE. Anti-CD20 chimeric monoclonal antibody (rituximab) for the treatment of recalcitrant, life-threatening pemphigus vulgaris with implications in the pathogenesis of the disorder. J Am Acad Dermatol 2002. https://doi.org/10.1067/mjd.2002.126273.
8. Ahmed AR, Kaveri S. Reversing autoimmunity combination of rituximab and IVIg. Front Immunol 2018;9:1189.
9. Wang HH, Liu CW, Li YC, et al. Efficacy of rituximab for pemphigus: a systematic review and meta-analysis of different regimens. Acta Derm Venereol 2015;95(8):928–32.
10. Almugairen N, Hospital V, Bedane C, et al. Assessment of the rate of long-term complete remission off therapy in patients with pemphigus treated with different regimens including medium- and high-dose corticosteroids. J Am Acad Dermatol 2013;69(4):583–8.
11. Kanwar AJ, Vinay K, Sawatkar GU, et al. Clinical and immunological outcomes of high- and low-dose rituximab treatments in patients with pemphigus: a randomized, comparative, observer-blinded study. Br J Dermatol 2014; 170(6):1341–9.
12. Ng CM, Bruno R, Combs D, et al. Population pharmacokinetics of rituximab (anti-CD20 monoclonal

antibody) in rheumatoid arthritis patients during a phase II clinical trial. J Clin Pharmacol 2005. https://doi.org/10.1177/0091270005277075.

13. Ahmed AR, Shetty S. A comprehensive analysis of treatment outcomes in patients with pemphigus vulgaris treated with rituximab. Autoimmun Rev 2015. https://doi.org/10.1016/j.autrev.2014.12.002.

14. Kim JH, Kim YH, Kim MR, et al. Clinical efficacy of different doses of rituximab in the treatment of pemphigus: a retrospective study of 27 patients. Br J Dermatol 2011;165(3):646–51.

15. Heelan K, Al-Mohammedi F, Smith MJ, et al. Durable remission of pemphigus with a fixed-dose rituximab protocol. JAMA Dermatol 2014. https://doi.org/10.1001/jamadermatol.2013.6739.

16. Gregoriou S, Giatrakou S, Theodoropoulos K, et al. Pilot study of 19 patients with severe pemphigus: prophylactic treatment with rituximab does not appear to be beneficial. Dermatology 2014; 228(2):158–65.

17. Strowd LC, Taylor SL, Jorizzo JL, et al. Therapeutic ladder for pemphigus vulgaris: emphasis on achieving complete remission. J Am Acad Dermatol 2011. https://doi.org/10.1016/j.jaad.2010.02.052.

18. Amber KT, Hertl M. An assessment of treatment history and its association with clinical outcomes and relapse in 155 pemphigus patients with response to a single cycle of rituximab. J Eur Acad Dermatol Venereol 2015. https://doi.org/10.1111/jdv.12678.

19. Keeley JM, Bevans SL, Jaleel T, et al. Rituximab and low dose oral immune modulating treatment to maintain a sustained response in severe pemphigus patients. J Dermatolog Treat 2018;1–6. https://doi.org/10.1080/09546634.2018.1510173.

20. Craythorne EE, Mufti G, Duvivier AW. Rituximab used as a first-line single agent in the treatment of pemphigus vulgaris. J Am Acad Dermatol 2011. https://doi.org/10.1016/j.jaad.2010.06.033.

21. Cho YT, Lee FY, Chu CY, et al. First-line combination therapy with rituximab and corticosteroids is effective and safe for pemphigus. Acta Derm Venereol 2014. https://doi.org/10.2340/00015555-1746.

22. Ingen-Housz-Oro S, Valeyrie-Allanore L, Cosnes A, et al. First-line treatment of pemphigus vulgaris with a combination of rituximab and high-potency topical corticosteroids. JAMA Dermatol 2015. https://doi.org/10.1001/jamadermatol.2014.2421.

23. Le Roux-Villet C, Prost-Squarcioni C, Alexandre M, et al. Rituximab for patients with refractory mucous membrane pemphigoid. Arch Dermatol 2011; 147(7):843–9.

24. Maley A, Warren M, Haberman I, et al. Rituximab combined with conventional therapy versus conventional therapy alone for the treatment of mucous membrane pemphigoid (MMP). J Am Acad Dermatol 2016. https://doi.org/10.1016/j.jaad.2016.01.020.

25. Heelan K, Walsh S, Shear NH. Treatment of mucous membrane pemphigoid with rituximab. J Am Acad Dermatol 2013. https://doi.org/10.1016/j.jaad.2013.01.046.

26. Schmidt E, Seitz CS, Benoit S, et al. Rituximab in autoimmune bullous diseases: mixed responses and adverse effects. Br J Dermatol 2007. https://doi.org/10.1111/j.1365-2133.2006.07646.x.

27. Hall RP, Streilein RD, Hannah DL, et al. Association of serum b-cell activating factor level and proportion of memory and transitional B cells with clinical response after rituximab treatment of bullous pemphigoid patients. J Invest Dermatol 2013. https://doi.org/10.1038/jid.2013.236.

28. Taverna JA, Lerner A, Bhawan J, et al. Successful adjuvant treatment of recalcitrant mucous membrane pemphigoid with anti-CD20 antibody rituximab. J Drugs Dermatol 2007;6(7):731–2.

29. Wollina U, Koch A, Hansel G. Rituximab therapy of recalcitrant bullous dermatoses. J Dermatol Case Rep 2008. https://doi.org/10.3315/jdcr.2008.1007.

30. Schumann T, Schmidt E, Booken N, et al. Successful treatment of mucous membrane pemphigoid with the anti-CD-20 antibody rituximab. Acta Derm Venereol 2009. https://doi.org/10.2340/00015555-0560.

31. Lourari S, Herve C, Doffoel-Hantz V, et al. Bullous and mucous membrane pemphigoid show a mixed response to rituximab: experience in seven patients. J Eur Acad Dermatol Venereol 2011. https://doi.org/10.1111/j.1468-3083.2010.03889.x.

32. Kasperkiewicz M, Shimanovich I, Ludwig RJ, et al. Rituximab for treatment-refractory pemphigus and pemphigoid: a case series of 17 patients. J Am Acad Dermatol 2011. https://doi.org/10.1016/j.jaad.2010.07.032.

33. Rübsam A, Stefaniak R, Worm M, et al. Rituximab preserves vision in ocular mucous membrane pemphigoid. Expert Opin Biol Ther 2015. https://doi.org/10.1517/14712598.2015.1046833.

34. Cho YT, Chu CY, Wang LF. First-line combination therapy with rituximab and corticosteroids provides a high complete remission rate in moderate-to-severe bullous pemphigoid. Br J Dermatol 2015. https://doi.org/10.1111/bjd.13633.

35. Bevans SL, Sami N. The use of rituximab in treatment of epidermolysis bullosa acquisita: three new cases and a review of the literature. Dermatol Ther 2018; e12726. https://doi.org/10.1111/dth.12726.

36. Cianchini G, Masini C, Lupi F, et al. Severe persistent pemphigoid gestationis: long-term remission with rituximab. Br J Dermatol 2007. https://doi.org/10.1111/j.1365-2133.2007.07982.x.

37. Tourte M, Brunet-Possenti F, Mignot S, et al. Pemphigoid gestationis: a successful preventive

treatment by rituximab. J Eur Acad Dermatol Venereol 2017. https://doi.org/10.1111/jdv.13962.

38. Albers LN, Zone JJ, Stoff BK, et al. Rituximab treatment for recalcitrant dermatitis herpetiformis. JAMA Dermatol 2017. https://doi.org/10.1001/jamadermatol.2016.4676.

39. Shetty S, Ahmed a R. Treatment of bullous pemphigoid with rituximab: critical analysis of the current literature. J Drugs Dermatol 2013;12(6):672–7.

40. Schulze J, Bader P, Henke U, et al. Severe bullous pemphigoid in an infant- successful treatment with rituximab. Pediatr Dermatol 2008;25(4):462–5.

41. Vinay K, Kanwar AJ, Sawatkar GU, et al. Successful use of rituximab in the treatment of childhood and juvenile pemphigus. J Am Acad Dermatol 2014. https://doi.org/10.1016/j.jaad.2014.05.071.

42. Kincaid L, Weinstein M. Rituximab therapy for childhood pemphigus vulgaris. Pediatr Dermatol 2016;33(2):e61–4.

43. Fuertes I, Guilabert A, Mascaro JMJ, et al. Rituximab in childhood pemphigus vulgaris: a long-term follow-up case and review of the literature. Dermatology 2010. https://doi.org/10.1159/000287254.

44. Szabolcs P, Reese M, Yancey KB, et al. Combination treatment of bullous pemphigoid with anti-CD20 and anti-CD25 antibodies in a patient with chronic graft-versus-host disease. Bone Marrow Transplant 2002. https://doi.org/10.1038/sj.bmt.1703654.

45. Connelly EA, Aber C, Kleiner G, et al. Generalized erythrodermic pemphigus foliaceus in a child and its successful response to rituximab treatment. Pediatr Dermatol 2007. https://doi.org/10.1111/j.1525-1470.2007.00369.x.

46. Fuertes I, Luelmo J, Leal L, et al. Refractory childhood pemphigoid successfully treated with rituximab. Pediatr Dermatol 2013. https://doi.org/10.1111/pde.12057.

47. Aoyama Y, Nagasawa C, Nagai M, et al. Severe pemphigus vulgaris: successful combination therapy of plasmapheresis followed by intravenous high-dose immunoglobulin to prevent rebound increase in pathogenic IgG. Eur J Dermatol 2008. https://doi.org/10.1684/ejd.2008.0471.

48. Hattori Y, Takahashi T, Seishima M. Bullous pemphigoid successfully treated with a combination therapy of plasmapheresis followed by intravenous high dose immunoglobulin. Ther Apher Dial 2017. https://doi.org/10.1111/1744-9987.12536.

49. Shimanovich I, Nitschke M, Rose C, et al. Treatment of severe pemphigus with protein A immunoadsorption, rituximab and intravenous immunoglobulins. Br J Dermatol 2008. https://doi.org/10.1111/j.1365-2133.2007.08358.x.

50. Kamphausen I, Schulze F, Schmidt E, et al. Treatment of severe pemphigus vulgaris of the scalp with adjuvant rituximab and immunoadsorption.

Eur J Dermatol 2012. https://doi.org/10.1684/ejd.2012.1843.

51. Behzad M, Möbs C, Kneisel A, et al. Combined treatment with immunoadsorption and rituximab leads to fast and prolonged clinical remission in difficult-to-treat pemphigus vulgaris. Br J Dermatol 2012. https://doi.org/10.1111/j.1365-2133.2011.10732.x.

52. Kasperkiewicz M, Shimanovich I, Meier M, et al. Treatment of severe pemphigus with a combination of immunoadsorption, rituximab, pulsed dexamethasone and azathioprine/mycophenolate mofetil: a pilot study of 23 patients. Br J Dermatol 2012; 166(1):154–60.

53. Kolesnik M, Becker E, Reinhold D, et al. Treatment of severe autoimmune blistering skin diseases with combination of protein A immunoadsorption and rituximab: a protocol without initial high dose or pulse steroid medication. J Eur Acad Dermatol Venereol 2014. https://doi.org/10.1111/jdv.12175.

54. Ahmed AR, Spigelman Z, Cavacini LA, et al. Treatment of pemphigus vulgaris with rituximab and intravenous immune globulin. N Engl J Med 2006; 355(17):1772–9.

55. Feldman RJ, Christen WG, Ahmed AR. Comparison of immunological parameters in patients with pemphigus vulgaris following rituximab and IVIG therapy. Br J Dermatol 2012. https://doi.org/10.1111/j.1365-2133.2011.10658.x.

56. Ahmed AR, Nguyen T, Kaveri S, et al. First line treatment of pemphigus vulgaris with a novel protocol in patients with contraindications to systemic corticosteroids and immunosuppressive agents: preliminary retrospective study with a seven year follow-up. Int Immunopharmacol 2016. https://doi.org/10.1016/j.intimp.2016.02.013.

57. Hamadah I, Chisti MA, Haider M, et al. Rituximab/IVIG in pemphigus—a 10-year study with a long follow-up. J Dermatolog Treat 2018;1–6. https://doi.org/10.1080/09546634.2018.1484873.

58. Nguyen T, Ahmed AR. Positive clinical outcome in a patient with recalcitrant bullous pemphigoid treated with rituximab and intravenous immunoglobulin. Clin Exp Dermatol 2017. https://doi.org/10.1111/ced.13092.

59. Ahmed AR, Shetty S, Kaveri S, et al. Treatment of recalcitrant bullous pemphigoid (BP) with a novel protocol: a retrospective study with a 6-year follow-up. J Am Acad Dermatol 2016. https://doi.org/10.1016/j.jaad.2015.11.030.

60. Foster CS, Chang PY, Ahmed AR. Combination of rituximab and intravenous immunoglobulin for recalcitrant ocular cicatricial pemphigoid. a preliminary report. Ophthalmology 2010. https://doi.org/10.1016/j.ophtha.2009.09.049.

61. Steger B, Madhusudan S, Kaye SB, et al. Combined use of rituximab and intravenous immunoglobulin for severe autoimmune cicatricial conjunctivitis—an

interventional case series. Cornea 2016. https://doi.org/10.1097/ICO.0000000000001024.

62. Boulard C, Duvert Lehembre S, Picard-Dahan C, et al. Calculation of cut-off values based on the autoimmune bullous skin disorder intensity score (ABSIS) and pemphigus disease area index (PDAI) pemphigus scoring systems for defining moderate, significant and extensive types of pemphigus. Br J Dermatol 2016. https://doi.org/10.1111/bjd.14405.

63. Rahbar Z, Daneshpazhooh M, Mirshams-Shahshahani M, et al. Pemphigus disease activity measurements: pemphigus disease area index, autoimmune bullous skin disorder intensity score, and pemphigus vulgaris activity score. JAMA Dermatol 2014. https://doi.org/10.1001/jamadermatol.2013.8175.

64. Ormond M, McParland H, Donaldson ANA, et al. An Oral Disease Severity Score validated for use in oral pemphigus vulgaris. Br J Dermatol 2018. https://doi.org/10.1111/bjd.16265.

65. Zhao CY, Murrell DF. Outcome measures for autoimmune blistering diseases. J Dermatol 2015. https://doi.org/10.1111/1346-8138.12711.

66. Du FH, Mills EA, Mao-Draayer Y. Next-generation anti-CD20 monoclonal antibodies in autoimmune disease treatment. Auto Immun Highlights 2017; 8(1). https://doi.org/10.1007/s13317-017-0100-y.

67. Huang A, Madan RK, Levitt J. Future therapies for pemphigus vulgaris: rituximab and beyond. J Am Acad Dermatol 2016;74(4):746–53.

68. De A, Ansari A, Sharma N, et al. Shifting focus in the therapeutics of immunobullous disease. Indian J Dermatol 2017;62(3):282–90.

69. Negrea GO, Elstrom R, Allen SL, et al. Subcutaneous injections of low-dose veltuzumab (humanized anti-CD20 antibody) are safe and active in patients with indolent non-Hodgkin's lymphoma. Haematologica 2011;96(4):567–73.

70. Ellebrecht CT, Choi EJ, Allman DM, et al. Subcutaneous veltuzumab, a humanized anti-CD20 antibody, in the treatment of refractory pemphigus vulgaris. JAMA Dermatol 2014;150(12):1331–5.

71. Quattrocchi E, Østergaard M, Taylor PC, et al. Safety of repeated open-label treatment courses of intravenous ofatumumab, a human anti-CD20 monoclonal antibody, in rheumatoid arthritis: results from three clinical trials. PLoS One 2016;11(6). https://doi.org/10.1371/journal.pone.0157961.

72. Schneider P, MacKay F, Steiner V, et al. BAFF, a novel ligand of the tumor necrosis factor family, stimulates B cell growth. J Exp Med 1999; 189(11):1747–56.

73. Hahne M, Kataoka T, Schröter M, et al. APRIL, a new ligand of the tumor necrosis factor family, stimulates tumor cell growth. J Exp Med 1998;188(6): 1185–90.

74. Litinskiy MB, Nardelli B, Hilbert DM, et al. DCs induce CD40-independent immunoglobulin class switching through BLyS and APRIL. Nat Immunol 2002;3(9):822–9.

75. Bossen C, Schneider P. BAFF, APRIL and their receptors: structure, function and signaling. Semin Immunol 2006;18(5):263–75.

76. Tangye SG, Bryant VL, Cuss AK, et al. BAFF, APRIL and human B cell disorders. Semin Immunol 2006; 18(5):305–17.

77. Asashima N, Fujimoto M, Watanabe R, et al. Serum levels of BAFF are increased in bullous pemphigoid but not in pemphigus vulgaris. Br J Dermatol 2006;155(2):330–6.

78. Nagel A, Podstawa E, Eickmann M, et al. Rituximab mediates a strong elevation of B-Cell-activating factor associated with increased pathogen-specific IgG but not autoantibodies in pemphigus vulgaris. J Invest Dermatol 2009;129(9):2202–10.

79. Sinha AA, Hoffman MB, Janicke EC. Pemphigus vulgaris: approach to treatment. Eur J Dermatol 2014;25(2):103–13.

80. Ellebrecht CT, Bhoj VG, Nace A, et al. Reengineering chimeric antigen receptor T cells for targeted therapy of autoimmune disease. Science 2016; 353(6295):179–84.

81. Hertl M, Amagai M, Sundaram H, et al. Recognition of desmoglein 3 by autoreactive T cells in pemphigus vulgaris patients and normals. J Invest Dermatol 1998;110(1):62–6.

82. Chow S, Rizzo C, Ravitskiy L, et al. The role of T cells in cutaneous autoimmune disease. Autoimmunity 2005;38(4):303–17.

83. Aoki-Ota M, Kinoshita M, Ota T, et al. Tolerance induction by the blockade of CD40/CD154 interaction in pemphigus vulgaris mouse model. J Invest Dermatol 2006;126(1):105–13.

84. Takahashi H, Amagai M, Nishikawa T, et al. Novel system evaluating in vivo pathogenicity of desmoglein 3-reactive T cell clones using murine pemphigus vulgaris. J Immunol 2008;181(2):1526–35.

85. Anhalt G, Werth V, Strober B, et al. An open-label phase I clinical study to assess the safety of PI-0824 in patients with pemphigus vulgaris. J Invest Dermatol 2005;(125):1088.

86. Berkowitz P, Hu P, Liu Z, et al. Desmosome signaling: inhibition of p38MAPK prevents pemphigus vulgaris IgG-induced cytoskeleton reorganization. J Biol Chem 2005;280(25):23778–84.

87. Berkowitz P, Hu P, Warren S, et al. p38MAPK inhibition prevents disease in pemphigus vulgaris mice. Proc Natl Acad Sci U S A 2006;103(34):12855–60.

88. Yoshida K, Ishii K, Shimizu A, et al. Non-pathogenic pemphigus foliaceus (PF) IgG acts synergistically with a directly pathogenic PF IgG to increase blistering by p38MAPK-dependent desmoglein 1 clustering. J Dermatol Sci 2017;85(3):197–207.

89. Mao X, Sano Y, Park JM, et al. p38 MAPK activation is downstream of the loss of intercellular adhesion in pemphigus vulgaris. J Biol Chem 2011;286(2):1283–91.

90. Sweeney SE, Firestein GS. Mitogen activated protein kinase inhibitors: where are we now and where are we going? Ann Rheum Dis 2006;65. https://doi.org/10.1136/ard.2006.058388.

91. Outerbridge C, Davis D, White S, et al. A new treatment for autoimmune blistering diseases - the efficacy of the Bruton's tyrosine kinase inhibitor PRN473 in canine pemphigus foliaceus. J Am Acad Dermatol 2016;74(5):AB141.

92. Smith CIE, Berglöf A. X-linked agammaglobulinemia. In: Adam MP, Ardinger HH, Pagon RA, et al, editors. GeneReviews. Seattle (WA): University of Washington; 2001. Available at: https://www.ncbi.nlm.nih.gov/books/NBK1453/.

93. ClinicalTrials.gov A study of PRN1008 in adult patients with pemphigus vulgaris—full text view - ClinicalTrials.gov. Available at: https://clinicaltrials.gov/ct2/show/NCT02704429?cond=pemphigus&rank=10. Accessed February 23, 2018.

94. Lotti R, Shu E, Petrachi T, et al. Soluble Fas ligand is essential for blister formation in pemphigus. Front Immunol 2018;9. https://doi.org/10.3389/fimmu.2018.00370.

95. Baker K, Rath T, Pyzik M, et al. The role of FcRn in antigen presentation. Front Immunol 2014. https://doi.org/10.3389/fimmu.2014.00408.

96. Li N, Zhao M, Hilario-Vargas J, et al. Complete FcRn dependence for intravenous Ig therapy in autoimmune skin blistering diseases. J Clin Invest 2005. https://doi.org/10.1172/JCI24394.

97. Incorvaia C, Mauro M, Russello M, et al. Omalizumab, an anti-immunoglobulin E antibody: state of the art. Drug Des Devel Ther 2014;8:197–207.

98. Lin H, Boesel KM, Griffith DT, et al. Omalizumab rapidly decreases nasal allergic response and FcεRI on basophils. J Allergy Clin Immunol 2004;113(2):297–302.

99. Romano C, Sellitto A, De Fanis U, et al. Omalizumab for difficult-to-treat dermatological conditions: clinical and immunological features from a retrospective real-life experience. Clin Drug Investig 2015;35(3):159–68.

100. Van Beek N, Lüttmann N, Huebner F, et al. Correlation of serum levels of IgE autoantibodies against BP180 with bullous pemphigoid disease activity. JAMA Dermatol 2017;153(1):30–8.

101. van Beek N, Schulze FS, Zillikens D, et al. IgE-mediated mechanisms in bullous pemphigoid and other autoimmune bullous diseases. Expert Rev Clin Immunol 2016;12(3):267–77.

102. Yu KK, Crew AB, Messingham KAN, et al. Omalizumab therapy for bullous pemphigoid. J Am Acad Dermatol 2014;71(3):468–74.

103. London VA, Kim GH, Fairley JA, et al. Successful treatment of bullous pemphigoid with omalizumab. Arch Dermatol 2012;148(11):1241–3.

104. Balakirski G, Alkhateeb A, Merk HF, et al. Successful treatment of bullous pemphigoid with omalizumab as corticosteroid-sparing agent: report of two cases and review of literature. J Eur Acad Dermatol Venereol 2016;30(10):1778–82.

105. Yalcin AD, Genc GE, Celik B, et al. Anti-IgE monoclonal antibody (omalizumab) is effective in treating bullous pemphigoid and its effects on soluble CD200. Clin Lab 2014;60(3):523–4.

106. Fairley JA, Baum CL, Brandt DS, et al. Pathogenicity of IgE in autoimmunity: successful treatment of bullous pemphigoid with omalizumab. J Allergy Clin Immunol 2009;123(3):704–5.

107. Dufour C, Souillet AL, Chaneliere C, et al. Successful management of severe infant bullous pemphigoid with omalizumab. Br J Dermatol 2012;166(5):1140–2.

108. Bilgiç Temel A, Bassorgun CI, Akman-Karakaş A, et al. Successful treatment of a bullous pemphigoid patient with rituximab who was refractory to corticosteroid and omalizumab treatments. Case Rep Dermatol 2017;9(1):38–44.

109. Menzinger S, Kaya G, Schmidt E, et al. Biological and clinical response to omalizumab in a patient with bullous pemphigoid. Acta Derm Venereol 2018;98(2):284–6.

110. Efficacy and safety of omalizumab in bullous pemphigoid—full text view - ClinicalTrials.gov. Available at: https://clinicaltrials.gov/ct2/show/NCT00472030. Accessed September 5, 2018.

111. Ding C, Li J, Zhang X. Bertilimumab Cambridge Antibody Technology Group. Curr Opin Investig Drugs 2004;5(11):1213–8.

112. Günther C, Wozel G, Meurer M, et al. Up-regulation of CCL11 and CCL26 is associated with activated eosinophils in bullous pemphigoid. Clin Exp Immunol 2011;166(2):145–53.

113. Kridin K. Peripheral eosinophilia in bullous pemphigoid: prevalence and influence on the clinical manifestation. Br J Dermatol 2018. https://doi.org/10.1111/bjd.16679.

114. Amber KT, Valdebran M, Kridin K, et al. The role of eosinophils in bullous pemphigoid: a developing model of eosinophil pathogenicity in mucocutaneous disease. Front Med (Lausanne) 2018;5:201.

115. Mrowietz U, Morrison PJ, Suhrkamp I, et al. The pharmacokinetics of fumaric acid esters reveal their in vivo effects. Trends Pharmacol Sci 2018;39(1):1–12.

116. Linker RA, Lee DH, Ryan S, et al. Fumaric acid esters exert neuroprotective effects in neuroinflammation via activation of the Nrf2 antioxidant pathway. Brain 2011;134(3):678–92.

117. Kornberg MD, Bhargava P, Kim PM, et al. Dimethyl fumarate targets GAPDH and aerobic glycolysis to modulate immunity. Science 2018;360(6387):449–53.

118. Wannick M, Assmann JC, Vielhauer JF, et al. The immunometabolomic interface receptor hydroxycarboxylic acid receptor 2 mediates the therapeutic effects of dimethyl fumarate in autoantibody-induced skin inflammation. Front Immunol 2018;9. https://doi.org/10.3389/fimmu.2018.01890.

119. Müller S, Behnen M, Bieber K, et al. Dimethylfumarate impairs neutrophil functions. J Invest Dermatol 2016;136(1):117–26.

120. Sadik CD, Miyabe Y, Sezin T, et al. The critical role of C5a as an initiator of neutrophil-mediated autoimmune inflammation of the joint and skin. Semin Immunol 2018;37:21–9.

121. Sezin T, Krajewski M, Wutkowski A, et al. The leukotriene B4 and its receptor BLT1 act as critical drivers of neutrophil recruitment in murine bullous pemphigoid-like epidermolysis bullosa acquisita. J Invest Dermatol 2017;137(5):1104–13.

122. Shrestha L, Bolaender A, Patel HJ, et al. Heat shock protein (HSP) drug discovery and development: targeting heat shock proteins in disease. Curr Top Med Chem 2016;16(25):2753–64.

123. Tukaj S, Tiburzy B, Manz R, et al. Immunomodulatory effects of heat shock protein 90 inhibition on humoral immune responses. Exp Dermatol 2014;23(8):585–90.

124. Kasperkiewicz M, Müller R, Manz R, et al. Heat-shock protein 90 inhibition in autoimmunity to type VII collagen: evidence that nonmalignant plasma cells are not therapeutic targets. Blood 2011;117(23):6135–42.

125. Ludwig RJ. Signalling and targeted therapy of inflammatory cells in epidermolysis bullosa acquisita. Exp Dermatol 2017;26(12):1179–86.

126. Tukaj S, Kleszczyński K, Vafia K, et al. Aberrant expression and secretion of heat shock protein 90 in patients with bullous pemphigoid. PLoS One 2013;8(7). https://doi.org/10.1371/journal.pone.0070496.

127. Han JM, Kwon NH, Lee JY, et al. Identification of gp96 as a novel target for treatment of autoimmune disease in mice. PLoS One 2010;5(3). https://doi.org/10.1371/journal.pone.0009792.

128. Rice JW, Veal JM, Fadden RP, et al. Small molecule inhibitors of Hsp90 potently affect inflammatory disease pathways and exhibit activity in models of rheumatoid arthritis. Arthritis Rheum 2008;58(12):3765–75.

129. Puri KD, Gold MR. Selective inhibitors of phosphoinositide 3-kinase delta: modulators of B-cell function with potential for treating autoimmune inflammatory diseases and B-cell malignancies. Front Immunol 2012;3. https://doi.org/10.3389/fimmu.2012.00256.

130. Koga H, Kasprick A, López R, et al. Therapeutic effect of a novel phosphatidylinositol-3-kinase δ inhibitor in experimental epidermolysis bullosa acquisita. Front Immunol 2018;9. https://doi.org/10.3389/fimmu.2018.01558.

What's New in Genetic Skin Diseases

Callie R. Hill, BS[a], Amy Theos, MD[b],*

KEYWORDS

- Genodermatoses • Next-generation sequencing • Targeted therapeutics
- Tuberous sclerosis complex • Congenital ichthyoses • PIK3CA-related overgrowth spectrum
- Interferonopathies • Basal cell nevus syndrome

KEY POINTS

- Next-generation sequencing technology has accelerated the discovery of genes underlying both constitutive and mosaic cutaneous disorders.
- Ustekinumab is effective for CARD14-associated papulosquamous eruption, including familial pityriasis rubra pilaris.
- Small-molecule inhibitors of the PI3K/AKT/mTOR pathway are promising treatments for mosaic overgrowth syndromes.
- JAK inhibitors are effective for the treatment of type I interferonopathies.
- Vismodegib and other smoothened inhibitors may cause irreversible fusion of growth plates in pediatric patients.

INTRODUCTION

Since the completion of the Human Genome Project in 2003, discoveries in genetic skin diseases have accelerated at a rapid pace, primarily due to advances in DNA sequencing technology and informatics, namely, next-generation sequencing (NGS) techniques.[1] These advances have dramatically improved the ability to diagnose a diverse group of inherited skin diseases and simplify disease classification based on pathogenesis, highlighting relationships among diseases. This information has translated to an improved understanding of disease mechanisms at a molecular level, allowed new insights into the structure and function of skin, and identified new therapeutic options based on molecular targets. This article highlights some of these recent advances and how they might translate into novel therapies and improved care for patients with genetic skin diseases.

WHAT IS NEW IN MOLECULAR DIAGNOSTICS

NGS has found its way from research laboratories into dermatology clinics, available through commercial laboratories and university-based medical centers. NGS, also known as massive parallel sequencing, allows a rapid and cost-effective approach to sequencing the protein-coding regions (whole exome sequencing or WES) or the entire genome (whole genome sequencing or WGS).[2] The protein-coding regions comprise about 1% of the total genome, but contain 85% of the disease-causing mutations, making WES preferred over WGS due to lower cost and more rapid turnaround time.[3] WES and WGS are most useful for gene discovery and as a diagnostic tool for patients with unclear or complex phenotypes. Often, these patients have undergone extensive testing without a definitive diagnosis. A recent study from a clinical laboratory reported a 32% diagnostic yield using WES for dermatologic

Disclosure: The authors state no financial disclosures or conflicts of interest.
[a] University of Alabama at Birmingham School of Medicine, 1720 2nd Avenue South, Birmingham, AL 35294, USA; [b] Department of Dermatology, University of Alabama at Birmingham, 1940 Elmer J. Bissell Road, Birmingham, AL 35243, USA
* Corresponding author.
E-mail address: amy.theos@childrensal.org

phenotypes.[4] Another study demonstrated the utility of WES in a genetic skin disease clinic, where it was used to confirm a diagnosis in 7 consecutive patients.[5] The cost of WES is currently comparable to the cost of more traditional single gene tests and may be a more cost-effective approach in some patients.[4]

NGS has led to the development of comprehensive multigene panels, which allows parallel sequencing of a group of defined genes of interest in a cost-effective and timelier manner compared with traditional Sanger sequencing.[6] Multigene panels are most useful for disorders with high genetic heterogeneity and a known spectrum of genetic causes (eg, epidermolysis bullosa, ichthyosis, and RAS/MAPK pathway-related disorders).[7–9] NGS has also improved the ability to diagnose mosaic skin disorders, which is reviewed later in this article.

WHAT IS NEW IN TUBEROUS SCLEROSIS COMPLEX

Tuberous sclerosis complex (TSC) is a genetic disorder characterized by multiple hamartomas in the skin, brain, kidneys, heart, lungs, and eye. The last 5 years has brought several important advances that will impact the management of patients with TSC, including updated, more specific, diagnostic criteria, publication of the TREATMENT trial for facial angiofibromas, and the recognition that sun exposure may cause angiofibroma development.

Updated Diagnostic Criteria

An accurate diagnosis of TSC is fundamental to the implementation of appropriate treatment and medical surveillance. The 1998 diagnostic criteria were recently updated and include the following changes: (1) identification of a pathogenic mutation in TSC1 or TSC2 as sufficient for diagnosis regardless of clinical findings and (2) refinement of the nomenclature and clinical features (size or number) for several of the dermatologic criteria.[10]

The clinical manifestations of TSC are highly variable and age dependent, making an accurate diagnosis based on clinical criteria alone challenging. Molecular testing of TSC1 and TSC2 genes detects a pathogenic mutation in 75% to 90% of patients with TSC.[11] A positive test result is enough to confirm a definitive diagnosis of TSC in a patient, even if they do not fulfill diagnostic criteria; however, a negative genetic test does not exclude TSC. Genetic testing should be considered in patients with an unclear diagnosis, for at-risk family members, and for prenatal testing. A listing of laboratories that offer testing can be found through the Tuberous Sclerosis

Alliance (www.tsalliange.org/about-tsc/how-is-tsc-diagnosed/. Accessed September 15, 2018) or through the Genetic Testing Registry (www.ncbi.nlm.nih.gov/gtr. Accessed September 15, 2018). An unknown percentage, but estimated to be at least 15%, of sporadic TSC cases are due to somatic mosaicism, which would not be detected from traditional sequencing methods on a blood sample.[12] NGS techniques with high-depth reads are used now by some laboratories and have a higher sensitivity, partly because of the ability of this test to detect low-level mosaicism in blood and saliva.[13] Affected tissue (eg, biopsy of angiofibromas or hypopigmented macule) can be submitted for testing if mosaicism is suspected and blood testing is negative.

The dermatologic and dental lesions used in the 1998 diagnostic criteria were maintained in the new criteria with minor revisions to nomenclature, number, and size of lesions.[13] The major and minor features of TSC, with changes bolded, are summarized in **Box 1**. A definitive diagnosis of TSC can be made by the identification of a pathogenic TSC1 or TSC2 mutation or the presence of 2 major features or 1 major feature plus ≥2 minor features. A possible diagnosis can be made with the presence of 1 major or ≥2 minor features.

Mammalian Target of Rapamycin Inhibitors for the Management of Tuberous Sclerosis Complex–Associated Manifestations

TSC is caused by mutations in either TSC1 or TSC2 leading to activation of the mammalian target of rapamycin (mTOR) signaling pathway, resulting in cell growth, proliferation, angiogenesis, and tumor formation.[14] Many of the manifestations of TSC are caused by the constitutive activation of the mTOR signaling pathway.[15] Not surprisingly, targeted therapies with mTOR inhibitors have revolutionized the treatment of TSC. The Food and Drug Administration approved everolimus for treatment of subependymal giant cell astrocytomas in 2010 and for renal angiomyolipomas in 2012 and sirolimus for pulmonary lymphangiomyomatosis in 2015.[16] These medications are also being investigated for the treatment of TSC-associated seizures and TSC-associated neuropsychiatric disorders as well as skin manifestations.

Facial angiofibromas typically begin to appear in childhood, affect up to 75% of patients, and have the potential to cause disfigurement and distress to patients.[17] Interventions such as excision, laser therapy, and dermabrasion are effective, but not ideal because of concerns of scarring, pain, anesthesia risks, and recurrence. Recent studies have

Major features (2 major or 1 major plus ≥2 minor needed for definitive diagnosis)

- Hypomelanotic macules (**≥3, at least 5 mm in diameter; areas of poliosis may be included in the count of HMMs**)
- Angiofibromas (**≥3; childhood onset; if onset in adulthood, it is counted as a minor criterion and BHD or MEN1 should be considered**) or **fibrous cephalic plaque** (changed from forehead plaque to reflect that these plaques may occur on other parts of the face or scalp)
- **Ungual** (encompasses periungual and subungual) fibromas (≥2)
- Shagreen patch (**collagenomas only, excludes other connective tissue nevi**)
- Multiple retinal hamartomas
- Cortical dysplasias
- Subependymal nodules
- Subependymal giant cell astrocytoma
- Cardiac rhabdomyoma
- Lymphangioleiomyomatosis
- Renal angiomyolipomas (≥2)

Minor features

- Confetti skin lesions
- Dental enamel pits (≥3)
- **Intraoral** (changed from gingival to reflect occurrence on other mucosae) fibromas (≥2)
- Retinal achromic patch
- Multiple renal cysts
- Nonrenal hamartomas

Genetic criteria

Identification of a pathogenic mutation in TSC1 or TSC2 gene is sufficient for diagnosis

Abbreviations: BHD, Birt-Hogg-Dube syndrome; HMMs, hypomelanotic macules; MEN1, multiple endocrine neoplasia type 1.

Data from Northrup H, Krueger DA, International Tuberous Sclerosis Complex Consensus Group. Tuberous sclerosis complex diagnostic criteria update: recommendations of the 2012 International Tuberous Sclerosis Complex Consensus Conference. Pediatr Neurol 2013;49:243–54; and Teng JM, Cowen EW, Wataya-Kaneda M, et al. Dermatologic and dental aspects of the 2012 International Tuberous Sclerosis Complex Consensus Statements. JAMA Dermatol 2014;150:1095–101.

focused on the use of mTOR inhibitors as a noninvasive treatment option for facial angiofibromas. Studies of oral sirolimus, used for noncutaneous indications, have shown improvement in the appearance of angiofibromas, with a reduction in erythema, number, and size of lesions, along with subjective patient improvement.[18–20] One study found an average improvement of 25% to 50% in female patients with lymphangiomyomatosis treated with sirolimus.[19] The efficacy of oral everolimus on skin lesions has been prospectively evaluated as a secondary endpoint in 2 phase 3 trials, and the response rate was significantly higher compared with placebo in both studies.[21] Given concerns about adverse effects, oral mTOR inhibitors are currently reserved for patients whose internal disease warrants systemic treatment.

For patients not requiring systemic treatment, topical mTOR inhibitors may be a safe and effective option. Since the first report of the success of topical sirolimus ointment for recalcitrant facial angiofibromas,[22] numerous case reports, small case series, and one small randomized controlled trial have been published, and these are nicely summarized by Jozwiak and colleagues.[23] Koenig and colleagues[24] recently published results from the largest randomized controlled trial to date (TREATMENT) and showed that once-daily application of topical sirolimus 1% or 0.1% significantly improved the appearance of angiofibromas compared with placebo, with the 1% concentration superior to the 0.1% concentration at the end of the 6-month trial. Adverse effects were minimal and limited to skin irritation, and serum levels of sirolimus were undetectable in all participants. These findings support previous reports of the safety and efficacy of topical sirolimus. However, future studies are still needed to determine the optimal concentration and vehicle, long-term safety (as continuous treatment is necessary to maintain response), durability of response, and whether prophylactic or very early use of topical sirolimus in pediatric patients is helpful in preventing the onset or altering the severity of angiofibromas. Given the safety of topical treatment, it seems reasonable to initiate treatment when angiofibromas begin appearing. Topical sirolimus has also shown variable efficacy for other TSC-associated skin lesions, including hypopigmented macules, collagenomas, and ungual fibromas.[25,26]

Sun Protection Is Important for Patients with Tuberous Sclerosis Complex

Sun-protective measures, including avoidance of sun exposure and use of hats and sunscreen, are especially important for patients with TSC and may reduce the number and severity of facial angiofibromas. A recent study evaluating the somatic second-hit mutations occurring in TSC-associated tumors identified a large population of UV "signature" mutations (CC > TT) in facial angiofibromas, suggesting sunlight-induced DNA damage as a cause of these mutations and the development of facial angiofibromas.[27] Sun protection is also important for patients on topical or oral mTOR inhibitors. Recently, in a mouse model of solar simulated light (SSL)-induced skin carcinogenesis, topical sirolimus reduced skin cancer formation when applied after SSL, but increased tumor formation when applied during and after SSL.[16,28] Counseling on the importance of sun protection should be provided to all patients with TSC.

WHAT IS NEW IN THE INHERITED ICHTHYOSES

The inherited ichthyoses encompass a large, clinically and genetically heterogeneous group of keratinization disorders resulting from abnormal epidermal barrier function with resultant varying degrees of scaling. The ichthyoses are broadly divided into 2 groups: non-syndromic (skin only) and syndromic (skin plus other organ systems).[29] Since the first clinically based classification scheme for inherited ichthyoses was published in 2010, advances in molecular diagnostics have led to the discovery of many novel genes causing ichthyoses, newly described syndromes, and an improved understanding of the cellular and biochemical mechanisms of the epidermal lipid barrier.[30] Ultimately, it is hoped that this information will improve patient care and lead to the development of novel pathway-based therapies.

Ustekinumab Effective for Familial Pityriasis Rubra Pilaris Caused by CARD14 Mutations

Pityriasis rubra pilaris (PRP) type V or atypical juvenile PRP represents about 6.5% of PRP cases and is an autosomal-dominant condition characterized by generalized ichthyosiform dermatitis. Familial PRP has been notoriously difficult to treat with unreliable response to various therapies, including oral retinoids, phototherapy, methotrexate, and tumor necrosis factor-α (TNF-α) inhibitors.[31] Recently, it was discovered that familial PRP is the result of gain-of-function mutations in *CARD14*.[32] *CARD14* activates nuclear factor κB signaling, promoting cutaneous inflammation, in part through production of interleukins (IL) -17, -22, and -23.[33] Interestingly, similar mutations in *CARD14* were previously identified in familial cases of psoriasis, suggesting shared

pathophysiology between these diseases.[34] Ustekinumab, a monoclonal antibody directed against IL-12 and IL-23 and approved for the treatment of psoriasis, has been shown to be beneficial for the treatment of familial PRP. Most reported cases have had complete or near complete clearance on therapy, although higher and more frequent dosing regimens may be necessary.[33,35] Ustekinumab has also been used successfully to treat adult and juvenile sporadic PRP.[36–38] Other biologics with similar mechanisms of action, including guselkumab (IL-23 inhibitor), secukinumab (IL-17A inhibitor), and ixekizumab (IL-17 inhibitor), may also be effective for both familial and sporadic PRP. Clinical trials evaluating ixekizumab and secukinumab for the treatment of sporadic PRP are currently underway (www.clinicaltrials.gov. Accessed September 15, 2018).

Craiglow and colleagues[39] propose the term CARD14-associated papulosquamous eruption (CAPE) to describe a spectrum of patients with early-onset disease, often with overlapping features of both PRP and psoriasis, which may benefit from treatment with ustekinumab. This study evaluated 15 kindreds with *CARD14* mutations, many with a suspected diagnosis of familial PRP. The investigators found that most patients had disease onset before age 1, had prominent involvement of cheeks, chin, upper lip, and ears with notable sparing of infralabial region, and had a family history of PRP or psoriasis. Notably, although the patients had failed numerous prior therapies (including TNF inhibitors), 5 of 6 ustekinumab-treated patients had complete clearance, and the sixth patient had partial clearance. Demonstration of *CARD14* mutations through genetic testing in patients with familial or sporadic PRP or clinical features suggestive of CAPE would suggest a role for treatment with ustekinumab or similar biologic.

Biologics Is a Promising Treatment for Severe Forms of Ichthyoses That Share Interleukin-17/Interleukin-23 Skewing

The orphan forms of the severe ichthyoses include autosomal-recessive congenital ichthyosis (encompasses lamellar and congenital ichthyosiform erythroderma [CIE] phenotypes), epidermolytic ichthyosis (formerly epidermolytic hyperkeratosis or bullous CIE), and Netherton syndrome. There currently are no effective and safe therapies for these debilitating diseases. Paller and colleagues[40] hypothesized that the immune alterations in response to an abnormal epidermal barrier may play a role in disease progression, and therapies targeting the inflammatory component, as opposed to the hyperkeratosis, could be beneficial. Paller and colleagues demonstrated that these ichthyoses all show impressive T helper 17 (Th17)/IL-23 skewing, very similar to psoriasis. Importantly, the degree of Th17-dominant inflammation in the skin correlated with ichthyoses severity and inflammation. Similarly, these investigators found significantly elevated IL-17 and IL-22–producing T cells in the blood of patients with these ichthyoses; again this correlated with clinical severity.[41] These findings suggest that biologics that antagonize IL-17, IL-22, or IL-23 might be beneficial for patients with severe ichthyoses. There is an ongoing study evaluation the efficacy of secukinumab (IL-17A inhibitor) in patients with severe ichthyoses (www.clinicaltrials.gov. Accessed September 15, 2018).

Evidence that targeting the inflammation in ichthyotic disorders can improve not only the erythema and pruritus but also the scaling and barrier function was recently published.[42] Two patients with newly described syndromes, erythrokeratodermia-cardiomyopathy (EKC) and severe dermatitis, multiple allergies, metabolic wasting syndrome, caused by mutations in *DSP1* responded to treatment with ustekinumab. Both patients, who had failed numerous other therapies, had significant decreases in pruritus, erythema, scaling, and transepidermal water loss by 12 weeks. Notably, both patients, who were very short in stature, experienced accelerated growth, suggesting benefits of treatment beyond the skin. Before treatment, immunophenotyping of skin and blood was performed in the patient with EKC, which showed Th17/IL-23 skewing and increased levels of IL-17 and IL-22, similar to the other severe ichthyoses detailed above.

WHAT IS NEW IN MOSAIC SKIN DISORDERS

Genomic mosaicism is caused by a postzygotic mutational event that results in 2 or more genetically different cell populations arising in an individual. Mosaicism is readily apparent in cutaneous disorders as asymmetric or patchy, patterned skin lesions that often respect the midline. When mutations occur early in embryonic development and affect pluripotent cells, widespread multisystem disease can occur. With the advent of NGS techniques, the molecular basis of many of these mosaic syndromic disorders has been discovered (**Table 1**). This new information has identified pathways central to disease pathogenesis, revealing potential novel targets for therapy.[43]

Molecular Testing of Mosaic Skin Disorders

Because of the mosaic nature of the genetic mutation, routine testing from a blood sample is unlikely to be informative. Therefore, affected tissue is necessary, ideally along with an unaffected, or control sample, such as blood or saliva. NGS, either through WES, WGS, or targeted testing including only genes of interest, is more likely to demonstrate low-level mosaicism compared with traditional Sanger sequencing and is a useful tool for identifying mutations in patients with suspected mosaic syndromes.[6]

Repurposing Cancer Therapies for Mosaic Overgrowth Syndromes

Postzygotic activating mutations of genes in the PI3K/AKT/mTOR pathway cause a group of congenital overgrowth syndromes. These disorders include Proteus syndrome and PIK3CA-related overgrowth spectrum (PROS) that encompass many diverse disorders, including CLOVES syndrome (congenital lipomatous overgrowth, vascular malformations, keratinocytic epidermal nevi, and skeletal/spinal anomalies), MCAP syndrome (megalencephaly-capillary malformation-polymicrogyria; previously macrocephaly-capillary malformation syndrome), and Klippel-Trenaunay syndrome (KTS).[44] These syndromes share features of asymmetric overgrowth of one or more tissue types (eg, skin, adipose, muscle, nerve), frequent developmental delays, various congenital anomalies, benign neoplasm (eg, epidermal nevi, vascular malformations, connective tissue nevi), and a variable increased risk of malignancy. These conditions cause considerable morbidity and mortality, and no effective treatment options other than surgery or symptomatic therapies exist.

Proteus is caused by mutations in *AKT1*, and PROS is caused by mutations most commonly in *PIK3CA*.[45,46] A mutation in either of these oncogenes causes activation of the PI3K/AKT/mTOR pathway leading to uncontrolled cell growth. Dysregulation of the pathway has been implicated in many cancers; thus, several small molecule inhibitors targeting PI3K, AKT, and mTOR have been approved for the treatment of cancer, and many more are in clinical trials.[44] It is likely that these compounds may be repurposed as targeted therapies for segmental overgrowth conditions.

BYL719, an oral inhibitor of *PIK3CA*, was recently demonstrated to improve organ dysfunction in a cohort of 19 patients with PROS/CLOVES syndrome who had life-threatening complications. All patients experienced improvement in a wide range of manifestations, including reduction in the size of vascular tumors, reduced hemihypertrophy, reversal of scoliosis, and improvement in congestive heart failure and cognitive function.[47] Side effects were minimal, and all patients remain

Table 1
Recently discovered genetic mutations underlying mosaic skin disorders

Mosaic Syndrome	Gene(s)	Key Clinical Features
Overgrowth syndromes Proteus	AKT1[45]	Asymmetric, progressive overgrowth of various tissues, connective tissue nevi, epidermal nevi, vascular malformations
PROS (includes CLOVES, megalencephaly-capillary malformation syndrome)	PIK3CA[46]	Congenital lipomatous overgrowth, complex vascular malformations, epidermal nevi, scoliosis, digit anomalies, megalencephaly, polymicrogyria
Klippel-Trenaunay syndrome	PIK3CA[50]	Capillary-lymphatic-venous malformation of a limb, overgrowth of soft tissue/bone
Vascular syndromes Sturge-Weber syndrome	GNAQ[78]	Facial port-wine stain involving V1, leptomeningeal angiomatosis, seizures, glaucoma
Phakomatoses pigmentovascularis	GNAQ, GNA11[79]	Extensive dermal melanocytosis and capillary malformation, neurovascular and ocular anomalies, seizures, developmental delay
Nevus syndromes Schimmelpenning-Feuerstein-Mims syndrome (NS syndrome)	HRAS, KRAS[80,88]	Extensive linear NS, KEN, CNS structural defects, seizures, colobomas, rickets
Phakomatosis pigmentokeratotica	HRAS[89]	Extensive NS, KEN, papular nevus spilus
Cutaneous skeletal hypophosphatemia syndrome	HRAS, NRAS[90,91]	Extensive NS, KEN, CMN, hypophosphatemic rickets, elevated FGF23
Large congenital melanocytic nevus/multiple congenital nevi	NRAS[92]	Large CMN or multiple CMN, neurocutaneous melanosis, other CNS pathologic condition
Miscellaneous Encephalocraniocutaneous lipomatosis	FGFR1[93]	Hairless lipomatous nevi on scalp, ocular tumors, CNS lipomas, seizures developmental delay
Oculoectodermal syndrome	KRAS[94]	Aplasia cutis, ocular dermoids, jaw fibromas, granular cell granulomas

Abbreviations: CMN, congenital melanocytic nevus; CNS, central nervous system; KEN, keratinocytic epidermal nevus; NS, nevus sebaceous.

on treatment. Notably, 9 patients had previously been treated with sirolimus without benefit. ARQ 092, a pan-*AKT* inhibitor, has demonstrated efficacy in vitro for patients with Proteus and PROS,[48,49] and clinical trials are underway for patients with these disorders (www.clinicaltrials.gov. Accessed September 15, 2018).

Most patients with KTS have mutations in *PIK3CA*, as do many patients with isolated lymphatic and venous malformations, and may respond to similar PI3K/AKT/mTOR inhibition.[50] BEZ235, a PI3K inhibitor in combination with everolimus, an mTOR inhibitor, was recently demonstrated to restore normal endothelial cell proliferation in a mouse model with *PIK3CA*-induced vascular malformations.[51] Sirolimus has been shown to be efficacious for a variety of complicated vascular anomalies, and there is a single case report of a patient with KTS and life-threatening hemorrhage treated successfully with oral sirolimus.[52,53]

WHAT IS NEW IN AUTOINFLAMMATORY INTERFERONOPATHIES

Type 1 interferonopathies are a recently described group of autoinflammatory monogenic disorders characterized by an upregulation of type 1 interferon (INF) production, including INF-α and INF-β.[54] The interferonopathies include Aicardi-Goutieres syndrome (AGS), stimulator of IFN genes-associated vasculopathy with onset in infancy (SAVI), and chronic atypical neutrophilic dermatosis with lipodystrophy and elevated temperatures (CANDLE). These disorders typically present in infancy with fever, systemic inflammation, skin findings, and organ damage and have a high mortality.

Recognition of the cutaneous manifestations is important to the early diagnosis and treatment of these syndromes. The characteristic skin findings in each syndrome include (1) chilblain-like lesions sparing the face in AGS; (2) severe cutaneous vasculopathy affecting face (mid cheeks, nose, ears), fingers and toes, painful distal ulcers, and tissue infarcts, generalized pustular eruption in infancy, telangiectasias, and livedo reticularis in SAVI; and (3) annular neutrophil-rich urticarial plaques, panniculitis, periorbital erythema and swelling, and progressive lipodystrophy in CANDLE.[55] The diagnosis of these syndromes can be supported by finding increased INF-α in the serum and an up-regulation of type I INF-stimulated genes (INF signature) in the blood. The diagnosis can be confirmed through genetic analysis (www.ncbi. nlm.nih.gov/gtr/. Accessed September 15, 2018).[56]

Janus Kinase Inhibitors for the Treatment of Type 1 Interferonopathies

This group of disorders is caused by mutations in a variety of genes that lead to either enhanced stimulation or defective negative regulation of INF production through the Janus kinase (JAK)/STAT pathway.[57] The JAK inhibitors (JAKinibs) are a group of oral small molecules approved for the treatment of arthritic and myeloproliferative disorders. JAKinibs block INF-α/β–induced activation of JAK, thus preventing STAT1 phosphorylation and the expression of IFN-induced genes and the autoinflammatory loop.[58] JAKinibs were shown to reduce type I and type II INF signaling in CANDLE and SAVI patients in vitro, suggesting a potential role for ameliorating disease symptoms in these patients.[59] Through an open-label expanded access program, Sanchez and colleagues treated 18 patients with various interferonopathies (CANDLE, SAVI, AGS, and 3 undefined cases) with baricitinib, a JAK 1/2 inhibitor, and monitored disease symptoms, reduction in corticosteroid requirement, quality of life, and changes in the INF signature. Patients were treated for a mean of 3 years, and almost all patients (15/18) showed significant improvement in disease symptoms from baseline, a decrease or discontinuation of corticosteroids, and an improved quality of life. The most common side effects were infectious, including BK viremia.[59] This study supports the findings of earlier smaller studies using JAKinibs, ruxolitinib and tofacitinib, to successfully treat patients with SAVI and familial chilblain lupus, respectively.[60,61] The JAK inhibitors appear to offer an effective, disease-modifying treatment for this group of rare monogenic syndromes characterized by the upregulation of type I INF.

WHAT IS NEW IN BASAL CELL NEVUS SYNDROME

Basal cell nevus syndrome (BCNS), also known as Gorlin syndrome, is an autosomal-dominant disorder that results in multiple basal cell carcinomas (BCCs) at an early age, along with odontogenic keratocysts, skeletal abnormalities, palmar/plantar pits, calcification of falx cerebri, and medulloblastoma.[62] The genetic basis of this syndrome has been identified with causative mutations in several tumor suppressor genes encoding important elements in the hedgehog (Hh) signaling pathway, including PTCH1, PTCH2, and SUFU.[63] Standard surgical therapies for BCC are often not ideal in these patients because of the large numbers of BCCs and the resultant risk of significant disfigurement. An effective targeted medial therapy would be an attractive alternative to repeated surgical procedures.

Vismodegib in the Treatment of Basal Cell Nevus Syndrome

Aberrant activation of the Hh pathway is a key driver in the pathogenesis of both syndromic and sporadic BCCs.[64] In 2012, vismodegib, an SMO, a critical activator of the Hh pathway, was approved to treat inoperable, locally advanced, or metastatic BCC.[65–67] Patients with BCNS were included in these pivotal trials, and vismodegib was shown to significantly reduce BCC tumor burden in these patients demonstrated by the low number of new surgically eligible BCCs and the reduction in size of existing BCCs in patients on vismodegib compared with placebo.[64,65] Unfortunately, adverse effects, including muscle spasms, alopecia, weight loss, and dysgeusia, were bothersome enough that half of the patients in one study (14 of 26) receiving vismodegib discontinued study participation.[65] In an open-label 36-month extension trial, only 3 patients were able to complete 36 months of continuous therapy.[68] BCCs recurred during interruption, but shrunk again after treatment was restarted.

Intermittent Vismodegib Therapy for Basal Cell Nevus Syndrome May Be Effective and Better Tolerated

Yang and Dinehart proposed that intermittent vismodegib therapy might be an effective way to improve tolerability and compliance in patients with BCNS, while still decreasing BCC tumor burden.[69] Treatment with intermittent vismodegib was investigated in a recently published study evaluating 2 intermittent vismodegib dosing regimens (A: 12 weeks vismodegib, 3 cycles of 8 weeks placebo/12 weeks vismodegib; B: 24 weeks vismodegib, 3 cycles of 8 weeks placebo/8 weeks vismodegib) for BCCs (MIKIE) that included 85 patients with BCNS. Both dosing regimens improved BCC burden over the 73-week study period, and although the reported adverse events were comparable to other studies, fewer patients (23%) on intermittent therapy discontinued the study because of these effects.[70] Patients with BCNS will likely need lifelong therapy, and further study to identify optimal, intermittent dosing regimens for these patients is warranted.

Basal Cell Carcinomas in Basal Cell Nevus Syndrome Show Increased Genomic Stability

Resistance, often due to acquired SMO and other somatic mutations, to treatment with vismodegib had been reported in up to 61% of patients with sporadic BCCs.[71] Fortunately, drug resistance seems to be much less frequent in patients with BCNS, although it has been reported.[68,71,72] Two recent studies found that syndromic BCC harbor fewer somatic SMO mutations at baseline compared with sporadic BCC.[71,73] In addition, the study by Chiang and colleagues found that syndromic BCC have a significantly lower mutational load, fewer UV-signature mutations, and increased genomic stability. These findings might explain the lower occurrence of drug resistance in BCNS patients treated with vismodegib, as well as their relatively more indolent course compared with sporadic BCCs.[71]

Vismodegib Causes Irreversible Fusion of Growth Plates in Pediatric Patients

Although the median age of first BCC in BCNS is 20 years, multiple BCCs can occur in children and have been reported as early as the first year of life.[62] The tumors in children often appear as flesh-colored or pigmented pedunculated papules (acrochordon-like), which histologically show BCC.[74] The management of multiple BCC in children is challenging. There is limited evidence for the use of vismodegib in pediatric patients with BCNS, although it has been used to treat BCCs in a child with xeroderma pigmentosum.[75] One concern raised in preclinical animal trials was the effect it could have on bone growth. This concern was recently substantiated by a report of 3 children with medulloblastoma treated with vismodegib who developed widespread, irreversible growth plate fusions with resultant profound short stature that occurred after prolonged exposure to the drug (>140 days).[76] Similarly, this has also been reported in patients treated with a similar drug, sonidegib.[77] It appears that the rate of growth plate fusions might be as high as 50% in children treated with Hh inhibitors for 6 months and 100% treated for 12 months. This finding has resulted in the exclusion of skeletally immature patients (defined as girls ≤14 years

and boys ≤16 years) from clinical trials and an updated warning label.[76]

SUMMARY

The post-Human Genome Project era has resulted in the accelerated discovery of novel disease-causing mutations underlying inherited skin diseases; this is likely to continue at an unprecedented pace, supported by continually evolving sequencing technologies. These advances have dramatically improved the ability to diagnose a diverse group of genetic skin diseases and have simplified disease classification schemes based on pathogenesis, highlighting relationships among diseases. More importantly, this information has translated to an improved understanding of disease mechanisms at a molecular level, allowed new insights into the structure and function of skin, and identified new therapeutic options based on molecular targets. This article has highlighted just a few of these recent discoveries. In this era of rapid advances in genomic medicine, it is important that dermatologists keep abreast of these developments to better diagnose, counsel, and treat patients and families affected by genetic skin diseases.

REFERENCES

1. International Human Genome Sequencing Consortium. Finishing the euchromatic sequence of the human genome. Nature 2004;431:931–45.
2. Lai-Cheong JE, McGrath JA. Next-generation diagnostics for inherited skin disorders. J Invest Dermatol 2011;131:1971–3.
3. Kwon EKM, Basel D, Siegel D, et al. A review of next-generation genetic testing for the dermatologist. Pediatr Dermatol 2013;30:401–8.
4. Retterer K, Juusola J, Cho MT, et al. Clinical application of whole-exome sequencing across clinical indications. Genet Med 2016;18:696–704.
5. Takeichi T, Nanda A, Liu L, et al. Impact of next generation sequencing on diagnostics in a genetic skin disease clinic. Exp Dermatol 2013;22:825–31.
6. Schaffer JV. Molecular diagnostics in genodermatoses. Semin Cutan Med Surg 2012;31:211–20.
7. Lucky AW, Dagaonkar N, Lammers K, et al. A comprehensive next-generation sequencing assay for the diagnosis of epidermolysis bullosa. Pediatr Dermatol 2018;35:188–97.
8. Diociaiuti A, El Hachem M, Pisaneschi E, et al. Role of molecular testing in the multidisciplinary diagnostic approach of ichthyosis. Orphanet J Rare Dis 2016;11:4.
9. Justino A, Dias P, Joao Pina M, et al. Comprehensive massive parallel DNA sequencing strategy for the

genetic diagnosis of the neuro-cardio-facio-cutaneous syndromes. Eur J Hum Genet 2015;23: 347–53.

10. Northrup H, Krueger DA, International Tuberous Sclerosis Complex Consensus Group. Tuberous sclerosis complex diagnostic criteria update: recommendations of the 2012 International Tuberous Sclerosis Complex Consensus Conference. Pediatr Neurol 2013;49:243–54.

11. Kozlowski P, Roberts P, Dabora S, et al. Identification of 54 large deletions/duplications in TSC1 and TSC2 using MLPA, and genotype-phenotype correlations. Hum Genet 2007;121:389–400.

12. Tyburczy ME, Dies KA, Glass J, et al. Mosaic and intronic mutations in TSC1/TSC2 explain the majority of TSC patients with no mutation identified by conventional Testing. PLoS Genet 2015;11: e1005637.

13. Teng JM, Cowen EW, Wataya-Kaneda M, et al. Dermatologic and dental aspects of the 2012 International Tuberous Sclerosis Complex Consensus Statements. JAMA Dermatol 2014;150:1095–101.

14. Franz DN, Capal JK. mTOR inhibitors in the pharmacologic management of tuberous sclerosis complex and their potential role in other rare neurodevelopmental disorders. Orphanet J Rare Dis 2017;12:51.

15. DiMario FJ Jr, Sahin M, Ebrahimi-Fakhari D. Tuberous sclerosis complex. Pediatr Clin North Am 2015;62:633–48.

16. Darling TN. Topical sirolimus to treat tuberous sclerosis complex (TSC). JAMA Dermatol 2018;154: 761–2.

17. Northrup H, Koenig MK, Pearson DA, et al. In: Adam AP, Ardinger HH, Pagon RA, et al, editors. GeneReviews [Internet]. Seattle (WA): University of Washington, Seattle; 1993–2018 [updated July 12, 2018].

18. Hofbauer GF, Marcollo-Pini A, Corsenca A, et al. The mTOR inhibitor rapamycin significantly improves facial angiofibromas lesions in a patient with tuberous sclerosis. Br J Dermatol 2008;159:473–5.

19. Nathan N, Wang JA, Li S, et al. Improvement of tuberous sclerosis complex (TSC) skin tumors during long-term treatment with oral sirolimus. J Am Acad Dermatol 2015;73:802–8.

20. Dabora SL, Franz DN, Ashwal S, et al. Multicenter phase 2 trial of sirolimus for tuberous sclerosis: kidney angiomyolipomas and other tumors regress and VEGF-D levels decrease. PLoS One 2011;6:e23379.

21. Cardis MA, DeKlotz CMC. Cutaneous manifestations of tuberous sclerosis complex and the paediatrician's role. Arch Dis Child 2017;102:858–63.

22. Haemel AK, O'Brian AL, Teng JM. Topical rapamycin: a novel approach to facial angiofibromas in tuberous sclerosis. Arch Dermatol 2010;146:715–8.

23. Jozwiak S, Sadowski K, Kotulska K, et al. Topical use of mammalian target of rapamycin (mTOR) inhibitors in tuberous sclerosis complex – a comprehensive review of the literature. Pediatr Neurol 2016;61:21–7.

24. Koenig MK, Bell CS, Herbert AA, et al. Efficacy and safety of topical rapamycin in patients with facial angiofibromas secondary to tuberous sclerosis complex: the TREATMENT randomize clinical trial. JAMA Dermatol 2018;154:773–80.

25. Wataya-Kaneda M, Tanaka M, Yang L, et al. Clinical and histologic analysis of the efficacy of topical rapamycin therapy against hypomelanotic macules in tuberous sclerosis complex. JAMA Dermatol 2015;151:722–30.

26. Muzic JG, Kindle SA, Tollefson MM. Successful treatment of subungual fibromas of tuberous sclerosis with topical rapamycin. JAMA Dermatol 2014; 150:1024–5.

27. Tyburczy ME, Wang JA, Li S, et al. Sun exposure causes somatic-hit mutations and angiofibroma development in tuberous sclerosis complex. JAMA Dermatol 2014;150:1095–101.

28. Dickinson SE, Janda J, Criswell J, et al. Inhibition of Akt enhances the chemopreventive effects of topical rapamycin in mouse skin. Cancer Prev Res 2016;9: 215–24.

29. Oji V, Tadini G, Akiyama M, et al. Revised nomenclature and classification of inherited ichthyoses: results of the First Ichthyosis Consensus Conference in Soreze 2009. J Am Acad Dermatol 2010;63: 607–41.

30. Zaki T, Choate K. Recent advances in understanding inherited disorders of keratinization. F1000Res 2018;7 [pii:F1000 Faculty Rev-919].

31. Mercer JM, Pushpanthan C, Anandakrishnan C, et al. Familial pityriasis rubra pilaris: case report and review. J Cutan Med Surg 2013;17:226–32.

32. Fuchs-Telem D, Sarig O, van Steensel MA, et al. Familial pityriasis rubra pilaris is caused by mutations in CARD14. Am J Hum Genet 2012;91:163–70.

33. Lwin SM, Hsu CK, Liu L, et al. Beneficial effect of ustekinumab in familial pityriasis rubra pilaris with a new missense mutation in CARD14. Br J Dermatol 2018;178:969–72.

34. Jordan CT, Cao L, Roberson ED, et al. PSORS2 is due to mutations in CARD14. Am J Hum Genet 2012;90:784–95.

35. Eytan O, Sarig O, Sprecher E, et al. Clinical response to ustekinumab in familial pityriasis rubra pilaris caused by a novel mutation in CARD14. Br J Dermatol 2014;171:420–2.

36. Wohlrab J, Kreft B. Treatment of pityriasis rubra pilaris with ustekinumab. Br J Dermatol 2010;163:655–6.

37. Napolitano M, Lembo L, Fania L, et al. Ustekinumab treatment of pityriasis rubra pilaris: a report of five cases. J Dermatol 2018;45:202–6.

38. Bonomo L, Raja A, Tan K, et al. Successful treatment of juvenile pityriasis rubra pilaris with ustekinumab in a 7-year-old girl. JAAD Case Rep 2018;4:206–10.

39. Craiglow BG, Boyden LM, Hu R, et al. CARD14-associated papulosquamous eruption: a spectrum including features of psoriasis and pityriasis rubra pilaris. J Am Acad Dermatol 2018;79:487–94.

40. Paller AS, Renert-Yuval Y, Suprun M, et al. An IL-17-dominant immune profile is shared across the major orphan forms of ichthyoses. J Allergy Clin Immunol 2017;139:152–65.

41. Czarnowicki T, He H, Leonard A, et al. The major orphan forms of ichthyoses are characterized by systemic T-cell activation and Th-17/Tc-17/Th-22/Tc-22 polarization in blood. J Invest Dermatol 2018. https://doi.org/10.1016/j.jid.2018.03.1523.

42. Paller AS, Czarnowicki T, Renert-Yuval Y, et al. The spectrum of manifestations in desmoplakin gene (DSP) spectrim repeat 6 domain mutations: immunophenotyping and response to ustekinumab. J Am Acad Dermatol 2018;78:498–505.

43. Vahidnezhad H, Youssefian L, Uitto J. Klippel-Trenaunay syndrome belongs to the PIK3CA-related overgrowth spectrum (PROS). Exp Dermatol 2016;25:17–9.

44. di Blasio L, Puliafito A, Gagliardi PA, et al. PI3K/mTOR inhibition promotes the regression of experimental vascular malformations driven by PIK3CA-activating mutations. Cell Death Dis 2018;9(2):45.

45. Adams DA, Trenor CC III, Hammill AM, et al. Efficacy and safety of sirolimus in the treatment of complicated vascular anomalies. Pediatrics 2016;137(2):e20153257.

46. Bessis D, Vernhet H, Bigorre M, et al. Life-threatening cutaneous bleeding in childhood Klippel-Trenaunay syndrome treated with oral sirolimus. JAMA Dermatol 2016;152:1058–9.

47. Crow YJ. Type I interferonopathies: a novel set of inborn errors of immunity. Ann N Y Acad Sci 2011;1238:91–8.

48. Kim H, Sanchez GA, Goldbach-Mansky R. Insights from Mendelian interferonopathies: Comparison of CANDLE, SAVI with AGS, monogenic lupus. J Mol Med (Berl) 2016;94:1111–27.

49. Munoz J, Rodiere M, Jeremiah N, et al. Stimulator of interferon genes-associated vasculopathy with onset in infancy: a mimic of childhood granulomatosis with polyangitis. JAMA Dermatol 2015;151:872–7.

50. Crow YJ. Type 1 interferonopathies: mendelian type I interferon up-regulation. Curr Opin Immunol 2015;32:7–12.

51. Hoffman HM, Broderick L. JAK inhibitors in autoinflammation. J Clin Invest 2018;128:2760–2.

52. Sanchez GAM, Reinhardt A, Ramsey S, et al. JAK1/1 inhibition with baricitinib in the treatment of autoinflammatory interferonopathies. J Clin Invest 2018;128:3041–52.

53. Fremond ML, Rodero MP, Jeremiah N, et al. Efficacy of the Janus kinase 1/2 inhibitor ruxolitinib in the treatment of vasculopathy associated with TMEM173-activating mutations in 3 children. J Allergy Clin Immunol 2016;138:1752–5.

54. Konig N, Fiehn C, Wolf C, et al. Familial chilblain lupus due to a gain-of-function mutation in STING. Ann Rheum Dis 2017;76:468–72.

55. Fogel AL, Sarin KY, Teng JMC. Genetic diseases associated with an increased risk of skin cancer development in childhood. Curr Opin Pediatr 2017;29:426–33.

56. Bree AF, Sha MR, BCNS Colloquium Group. Consensus statement from the first international colloquium on basal cell nevus syndrome (BCNS). Am J Med Genet A 2011;155A:2091–7.

57. Chang AL, Arron ST, Migden MR, et al. Safety and efficacy of vismodegib in patients with basal cell carcinoma nevus syndrome: pooled analysis of two trials. Orphanet J Rare Dis 2016;11:120.

58. Tang JY, Mackay-Wiggan JM, Aszterbaum M, et al. Inhibiting the hedgehog pathway in patients with basal-cell nevus syndrome. N Engl J Med 2012;366:2180–8.

59. Sekulic A, Migden MR, Oro AE, et al. Efficacy and safety of vismodegib in advanced basal-cell carcinoma. N Engl J Med 2012;366:2171–9.

60. Chang AL, Solomon JA, Hainsworth JD, et al. Expanded access study of patients with advanced basal cell carcinoma treated with Hedgehog pathway inhibitor, vismodegib. J Am Acad Dermatol 2014;70:60–9.

61. Tang JY, Ally MS, Chanana AM, et al. Inhibition of the hedgehog pathway in patients with basal-cell nevus syndrome: final results from the multicentre, randomized, double-blind, placebo-controlled, phase 2 trial. Lancet Oncol 2016;17:1720–31.

62. Yang X, Dinehart SM. Intermittent vismodegib therapy in basal cell nevus syndrome. JAMA Dermatol 2016;152:223–4.

63. Dreno B, Kunstfeld R, Hauschild A, et al. Two intermittent vismodegib dosing regimens in patients with multiple basal-cell carcinomas (MIKIE): a randomized, regimen-controlled, double blind, phase 2 trial. Lancet Oncol 2017;18:404–12.

64. Chiang A, Jaiu PD, Batra P, et al. Genomic stability in syndromic basal cell carcinoma. J Invest Dermatol 2018;138:1044–51.

65. Sinx KAE, Roemen GMJM, van Zutven V, et al. Vismodegib-resistant basal cell carcinomas in basal cell nevus syndrome: clinical approach and genetic analysis. JAAD Case Rep 2018;4:408–11.

66. Bonilla X, Parmentier L, King B, et al. Genomic analysis identifies new drivers and progression pathways in skin basal cell carcinoma. Nat Genet 2016;48:398–406.

67. Chiritescu E, Maloney ME. Acrochordons as a presenting sign of nevoid basal cell carcinoma syndrome. J Am Acad Dermatol 2001;44:789–94.

68. Fife D, Laitinen MA, Myers DJ, et al. Vismodegib therapy for basal cell carcinoma in an 8-year-old Chinese boy with xeroderma pigmentosum. Pediatr Dermatol 2017;34:163–5.

69. Robinson GW, Kaste SC, Chemaitilly W, et al. Irreversible growth plate fusions in children with medulloblastoma treated with a targeted hedgehog pathway inhibitor. Oncotarget 2017;8:69295–302.

70. Kieran MW, Chisholm J, Casanova M, et al. Phase I study of oral sonidegib (LDE225) in pediatric brain and solid tumors and a phase II study in children and adults with relapsed medulloblastoma. Neuro Oncol 2017;19:1542–52.

71. Shirley MD, Tang H, Gallione CJ, et al. Sturge-Weber syndrome and port-wine stains caused by somatic mutation in GNAQ. N Engl J Med 2013;368:1971–9.

72. Thomas AC, Zeng A, Riviere JB, et al. Mosaic activating mutations in GNA11 and GNAQ are associated with phakomatosis pigmentovascularis and extensive dermal melanocytosis. J Invest Dermatol 2016;136:770–8.

73. Asch S, Sugarman JL. Epidermal nevus syndromes: new insights into whorls and swirls. Pediatr Dermatol 2018;35:21–9.

74. Happle R. The categories of cutaneous mosaicism: a proposed classification. Am J Med Genet A 2016;170A:452–9.

75. Groesser L, Herschberger E, Sagrera A, et al. Phacomatosis pigmentokeratotica is caused by a postzygotic HRAS mutation in a multipotent progenitor cell. J Invest Dermatol 2013;133:1998–2003.

76. Lim YH, Ovejero D, Sugarman JS, et al. Multilineage somatic activating mutations in HRAS and NRAS cause mosaic cutaneous and skeletal lesions, elevated FGF23 and hypophosphatemia. Hum Mol Genet 2014;23:397–407.

77. Lim YH, Ovejero D, Derrick KM, et al. Cutaneous skeletal hypophosphatemia syndrome (CSHS) is a multilineage somatic mosaic RASopathy. J Am Acad Dermatol 2015;75:420–7.

78. Kinsler VA, Thomas AC, Ishida M, et al. Multiple congenital melanocytic nevi and neurocutaneous melanosis are caused by postzygotic mutations in codon 61 or NRAS. J Invest Dermatol 2013;133:2229–36.

79. Bennett JT, Alcantara D, Tetrault M, et al. Mosaic activating mutations in FGFR1 cause encephalocraniocutaneous lipomatosis. Am J Hum Genet 2016;98:579–87.

80. Peacock JD, Dykema KJ, Toriello HV, et al. Oculoectodermal syndrome is a mosaic RASopathy associated with KRAS alterations. Am J Med Genet A 2015;167:1429–35.

Moving?

Make sure your subscription moves with you!

To notify us of your new address, find your **Clinics Account Number** (located on your mailing label above your name), and contact customer service at:

Email: journalscustomerservice-usa@elsevier.com

800-654-2452 (subscribers in the U.S. & Canada)
314-447-8871 (subscribers outside of the U.S. & Canada)

Fax number: 314-447-8029

Elsevier Health Sciences Division
Subscription Customer Service
3251 Riverport Lane
Maryland Heights, MO 63043

*To ensure uninterrupted delivery of your subscription, please notify us at least 4 weeks in advance of move.

ELSEVIER